T0202037

Adjustment Disorder

Adjustment Disorder
From Controversy to Clinical Practice

Patricia Casey

Consultant Psychiatrist, Mater Misericordiae
University Hospital, Dublin, Ireland;

Emeritus Professor of Psychiatry,
University College Dublin, Ireland;

Editor, *BJPsych Advances*, Royal College
of Psychiatrists, London, UK

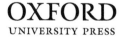

OXFORD
UNIVERSITY PRESS

OXFORD

UNIVERSITY PRESS

Great Clarendon Street, Oxford, OX2 6DP,
United Kingdom

Oxford University Press is a department of the University of Oxford.
It furthers the University's objective of excellence in research, scholarship,
and education by publishing worldwide. Oxford is a registered trade mark of
Oxford University Press in the UK and in certain other countries

First Edition published in 2018

Impression: 1

Published in the United States of America by Oxford University Press
198 Madison Avenue, New York, NY 10016, United States of America

British Library Cataloguing in Publication Data

Data available

Library of Congress Control Number: 2017959076

ISBN 978–0–19–878621–4

Printed and bound by
CPI Group (UK) Ltd, Croydon, CR0 4YY

To the memory of my beloved son Gavan McGuiggan, who showed endurance, wit, and an indomitable spirit in coping with a long and serious illness.

Contents

Contributors

Elspeth Bradley
Associate Professor, Department of Psychiatry, University of Toronto, Toronto, ON, Canada

Patricia Casey
Consultant Psychiatrist, Mater Misericordiae University Hospital, Dublin, Ireland; Emeritus Professor of Psychiatry, University College Dublin, Ireland; Editor, *BJPsych Advances*, Royal College of Psychiatrists, London, UK

Anne Doherty
Consultant Liaison Psychiatrist, Galway University Hospitals, Galway, Ireland; Honorary Senior Lecturer in Psychiatry, National University of Ireland, Galway, Ireland

Sheila Hollins
Emeritus Professor of Psychiatry of Learning Disability, St George's, University of London, UK

Marika Korossy
Former Librarian, Surrey Place Centre, Toronto, ON, Canada

Andrew Levitas
Professor of Psychiatry, Rowan University, School of Medicine, Medical Director, Center of Excellence for the Mental Health Treatment of Persons with Intellectual Disabilities, Glassboro, NJ, USA

Aisling Mulligan
Clinical Associate Professor, Department of Child and Adolescent Psychiatry, University College Dublin, Ireland; Dublin North City and County Child and Adolescent Mental Health Service, Health Services Executive, Dublin, Ireland

Geoffrey Reid
Consultant Psychiatrist, Military Medical Personnel (MMP), London, UK

Keith Rix
Visiting Professor of Medical Jurisprudence, University of Chester, UK; Honorary Consultant Forensic Psychiatrist, Norfolk and Suffolk NHS Foundation Trust, UK

Chapter 1

History of the concept of adjustment disorders

Patricia Casey

Stress and its history

The history of stress begins with Hippocrates, who wrote that disease was not only suffering (*pathos*) but also toil (*ponos*) as the body tried to restore normality. Stress-related psychological symptoms were also mentioned by the eleventh-century Islamic philosopher and doctor, Avicenna. The word 'stress' was used for centuries in physics to depict elasticity, the property of a material that allows it to resume its original size and shape after it has been subjected to an external force. Hooke's law (1658) states that the magnitude of an external force, or stress, produces a proportional amount of deformation, or strain, in a malleable metal, an effect also seen in response to psychological stress. Hans Selye, a Hungarian doctor who worked in Canada, is the name most associated with 'stress', the term used to describe the non-specific response of the organism to threats. Although he was working on this at McGill University from the 1930s onwards, the concept of stress did not come to widespread attention until the 1970s. In his early work that Seyle published as a letter in *Nature*, he described the 'General Adaptation Syndrome' (1), which represented the response of the body to demands placed upon it. He later renamed this 'stress'. He later showed that a stress response occurred whether the trigger was negative or positive: the former he called 'distress' and the latter 'eustress', which has the capacity to enhance functioning. He was influenced in this by the work of Lennart Levi (2), Emeritus Professor of Psychosocial Medicine at the Karolinska Institute in Sweden.

Selye also identified the hypothalamo-pituitary axis as the hormonal system that was responsible for the stress response, and he identified three phases relating to this. The first is the *alarm* phase, in which the body responds to a stressor with the 'fight-or-flight' response when the sympathetic nervous system is activated; the second, or *resistance*, phase is marked by attempts to restore normal functioning or homeostasis through the activity of the parasympathetic nervous system; and the third, or *exhaustion*, phase occurs when the stressor continues and exhausts the body's capacity to return to normal physiological functioning, resulting in pathology. Later in his work he used the word 'stressor' to describe the trigger or event to which the system had to adapt, and 'stress' to describe the response to an event. This was the result of an observation that in his earlier development of the concept, the word 'stress' represented both the response and the trigger, a position that was tautological and illogical.

From stress to adjustment disorder

Selye had always emphasized that the stressors could be physical, chemical, or psychological. Whether as a result of his continuing research and the foundation of the International Institute of Stress in 1975, or simply by coincidence, the realization that abnormal, time-limited, psychological stress responses did occur first received official recognition when the term 'adjustment disorder' was introduced into the ICD-9 (International Classification of Diseases, Ninth Revision) in 1978 (3) and the DSM-III (*Diagnostic and Statistical Manual of Mental Disorders, Third Edition*) in 1980 (4).

Adjustment disorder (AD) is a psychiatric condition that arises in response to a stressful event or situation. It resolves spontaneously once the stressor is removed or when a new level of adaptation is reached. AD is unusual among psychiatric disorders because it is one of the few syndromes in the current classifications to link aetiology with diagnosis. In this, it resembles bereavement, acute stress disorder (ASD), and post-traumatic stress disorder (PTSD). This group of conditions are collectively termed the 'Trauma and Stress-related Disorders' and they are the exception in being classified by their aetiology since both DSM-5 (5) and ICD-10 (6) explicitly state that they are neutral in this regard. This is why words such as 'neurotic' no longer appear in these manuals as this would imply a particular type of aetiology stemming from internal conflicts.

AD and its precursors in the International Classification of Diseases

Historically, AD is broadly similar in the DSM and the ICD classifications. The closest equivalent to AD in the seventh edition of the ICD (7) were the terms 'anxiety reaction' NOS as one of the conditions in the category Anxiety Reaction without Mention of Somatic Symptoms. Another is 'reactive depression' and 'psychogenic depression' in the category Neurotic-depressive Reaction.

ICD-8 (8) introduced the term 'transient situational disturbance', changed it to 'adjustment reaction' with the publication of ICD-9 in 1978, and subsequently to 'adjustment disorder' in ICD-10 (6). This term is retained in ICD-11 (9).

Seven subtypes are identified in ICD-10 (see Box 1.1), among them the specifiers 'brief' and 'prolonged' depressive reactions. The definition in ICD-10 specifically excludes events that are catastrophic or unusual.

The ICD-10 criteria for AD are described in Box 1.1:

Box 1.1 Summary of criteria for Adjustment Disorders in ICD-10 (F43.20)

A. The individual must have experienced an identifiable psychosocial stressor, not of an unusual or catastrophic type, within 1 month of the onset of symptoms.

B. The symptoms or behaviour disturbance resemble those found in any of the affective disorders (except for delusions and hallucinations), any disorders in F4 (neurotic, stress related and somatoform disorders), and conduct disorders, but the criteria of an individual disorder are not met.

Symptoms may be variable in both form and severity.

The predominant feature of the symptoms may be specified by the use of a fifth character:

(continued)

Box 1.1 (Continued)

F43.20 Brief depressive reaction. A transient mild depressive state not exceeding 1 month;

F43.21 Prolonged depressive reaction. A mild depressive state occurring in response to a prolonged exposure to a stressful situation not exceeding 2 years;

F43.22 Mixed anxiety and depressive reaction. Both of these symptoms are prominent, but at levels no greater than specified in mixed anxiety and depressive disorder (F41.20) or other mixed anxiety disorders (F41.30);

F43.23 With predominant disturbance of other emotions. These comprise several types of emotion, such as anxiety, depression, worry, tensions, and anger. Symptoms of anxiety and depression may meet the criteria for mixed anxiety and depressive disorder (F41.20) or other mixed anxiety disorders (F41.30), but they do not reach the threshold for other more specific depressive or anxiety disorders. This category should also be used for reactions in children in which regressive behaviour such as bedwetting or thumb-sucking is also present;

F43.24 With predominant disturbance of conduct. The main disturbance is one involving conduct, e.g. an adolescent grief reaction leading to aggressive or other dissocial behaviour;

F43.25 With mixed disturbance of emotions and conduct. Both emotional symptoms and disturbances of conduct are prominent features;

F43.28 With other specified predominant symptoms.

C. The symptoms do not persist for more than 6 months, except when the stressor is prolonged.

Source: data from ICD-10: The ICD-10 Classification of Mental and Behavioural Disorders: Clinical Descriptions and Diagnostic Guidelines, Copyright (1992), WHO Organization

AD and its precursors in the *Diagnostic and Statistical Manual of Mental Disorders*

DSM-I (10) introduced the category of transient situational personality disorders, a term broadly similar to AD. This included subtypes such as gross stress reaction; adult situational reactions; and adjustment reaction of infancy, of childhood, of adolescence, of late life, and other.

DSM-II (11) refined the name and called it acute situational disorder to encapsulate any transient reaction to overwhelming stress in an individual without any apparent underlying mental disorder. It could be of any severity, and included psychotic reactions. It continued to use the lifespan subtypes while eliminating the gross stress reaction and adult situational reactions listed in DSM-I (10). Although it was supposed not to be diagnosed when another major disorder was present, this dictum was often ignored.

DSM-III (12) changed to the new term 'adjustment disorder' and eliminated the lifespan terminologies, replacing them with subtypes based on the main mood and/or behavioural features. The subtypes included the depressive, the anxious, the mixed anxiety and depression, the disturbance of conduct, and the disturbance of conduct and emotions groups, and/or with work inhibition, withdrawal, and atypical features. The revision of DSM III-R in 1987 (13) made further modifications that included a specifier of 6 months' duration and a subtype 'with physical symptoms'.

DSM-IV (14) removed the subtypes relating to inhibition, withdrawal, atypical features and physical symptoms, and added a chronic specifier. The specifiers state that AD many be acute (lasting less than 6 months) or chronic (prolonged if the stressor or its consequences continues), but may last no longer than 6 months after cessation of the stressor.

Now, DSM-5 (5) has made no change to the criteria themselves, but has moved AD from being an orphaned category to its inclusion in the Trauma and Stress-related Disorders grouping. As with previous editions of DSM, a diagnosis of AD requires clinically significant symptoms or impairment, and it cannot be diagnosed when the threshold for another disorder is reached. Neither can it be diagnosed when the person is bereaved.

The DSM-5 criteria for adjustment disorder are described in Box 1.2.

The subtypes are identical in DSM-IV (14) and DSM-5 (5). Table 1.1 compares the subtypes in both classifications.

Box 1.2 Summary of criteria for adjustment disorders in DSM-5

A. The individual develops emotional or behavioural symptoms in response to an identifiable stressor(s) occurring within 3 months of the onset of the stressor(s).

B. These symptoms or behaviours are clinically significant, as evidenced by one or both of the following:

1. Marked distress that is out of proportion to the severity or intensity of the stressor. This must take into account the external context and the cultural factors that might influence symptom severity and presentation;

2. Significant impairment in social, occupational, and/or other areas of functioning.

C. The stress-related disturbance does not meet the criteria for another mental disorder and the symptoms do not represent an exacerbation of a pre-existing mental disorder.

D. The symptoms do not represent normal bereavement.

E. Once the stressor or its consequences have terminated, the symptoms do not persist for more than an additional 6 months.

Source: data from the Diagnostic and Statistical Manual of Mental Disorders, Fifth Edition, DSM-5, Copyright (2013), American Psychiatric Association

In both the current DSM and ICD classifications, the diagnosis cannot be made when the threshold for another condition is reached. So when the duration or symptom numbers are met for a person experiencing distress symptoms, the diagnosis of AD is overtaken by another related disorder—most commonly, major depressive disorder (MDD) or generalized anxiety disorder (GAD). Thus, in both it is a subthreshold disorder.

For all diagnoses in DSM-5, including AD, the symptoms must be clinically significant. They must also cause distress *and* impairment in ICD-10, while distress *or* impairment is required in DSM-5. This suggests that the threshold for making a psychiatric diagnosis is lower in the DSM classification than in the ICD classification. The issue of thresholds will be discussed in greater detail in Box 1.3 and in Chapter 3, pp. 44–7.

Table 1.1 Subtypes of AD in DSM-IV, DSM-5, and ICD-10

DSM-IV/DSM-5	ICD-10
AD with depressed mood (309.0)	AD with brief depressive reaction F43.20
	AD with prolonged depressive reaction F43.21
AD with anxiety (309.24)	AD with mixed anxiety and depressive
AD with depression and anxiety (309.28)	reaction F43.22
AD with disturbance of conduct (309.3)	AD with predominant disturbance of other emotions F43.23
	AD with predominant disturbance of conduct F43.24
AD with disturbance of emotion and conduct (309.4)	AD with mixed disturbance of emotions and conduct F43.25
AD unspecified (309.9)	AD with other specified predominant symptoms F43.26

Source: data from Diagnostic and Statistical Manual of Mental Disorders, Fourth Edition, DSM-IV, Copyright (1994), American Psychiatric Association; Diagnostic and Statistical Manual of Mental Disorders, Fifth Edition, DSM-5, Copyright (2013), American Psychiatric Association; ICD-10: The ICD-10 Classification of Mental and Behavioural Disorders: Clinical Descriptions and Diagnostic Guidelines, Copyright (1992), WHO Organization

Evolution to full-threshold status and the ICD-11 proposals

While DSM-5 has moved AD from being a stand-alone category into the Trauma and Stress-related Disorders grouping, its status as a full-threshold disorder is still not recognized, and so the diagnosis is superseded when the threshold for another disorder is reached. The issue of thresholds is highlighted in the example in Box 1.3.

ICD-10 currently includes AD in the Trauma and Stress-related Disorders grouping, and as with DSM-5, it is regarded as a subthreshold diagnosis. The proposal for ICD-11 (9) takes a very different approach to ICD-10 and DSM-5 by recognizing it as a full-threshold disorder analogous to MDD or GAD. This, along with other changes to the criteria for ICD-11, makes the proposal radical.

Radical ICD-11 proposal

The proposed operational definition for AD in ICD-11 is as follows:

1. Presence of an identifiable stressor(s) or life change(s);

2. Occurrence of symptoms of preoccupation related to the stressor in the form of at least one of the following:

(2a) significant excessive worry about the stressor

(2b) recurrent and distressing thoughts about the stressor

(2c) constant rumination about the implications of the stressor;

3. Failure to adapt, as manifested by either (2a) or (2b) or both, that significantly interferes with everyday functioning:

    (3a) difficulties concentrating

    (3b) sleep disturbance resulting in performance problems at work or at school;

4. Symptoms emerge within a month of the onset of the stressor(s) and tend to resolve in 6 months unless the stressor persists for a longer duration;

5. Symptoms must be associated with significant distress and significant impairment in personal, family, social, educational, occupational, or other important areas of functioning.

The subtypes of AD recognized in DSM-5 will be eliminated in ICD-11 as these are not well validated (15), but the acute and chronic specifiers will be retained.

These criteria are still at the discussion stage, but if they are accepted for inclusion in ICD-11, there will be more differences than similarities between AD as characterized in DSM-5 and as characterized in ICD-11. Table 1.2 describes the differences between the two classifications.

Table 1.2 Comparison of criteria in ICD-11 and DSM-5

Classification	Onset after stressor	Diagnostic criteria	Symptoms /impairment	Subtypes	Threshold status
ICD-11	Up to 1 month	Specific symptoms	Both (usually)	Eliminated	Full threshold
DSM-5	Up to 3 months	Non-specific symptoms	One or the other	Seven subtypes	Subthreshold

Source: data from ICD-11: The ICD-11 International Classification of Diseases, Copyright (2018), WHO Organization; Diagnostic and Statistical Manual of Mental Disorders, Fifth Edition, DSM-5, Copyright (2013), American Psychiatric Association

Box 1.3 Case vignette 1: Adjustment disorder and the threshold issue

Ms A is 24 and she works as a secretary in an accountant's office. She often feels undermined by her manager. It comes to a head when she is publicly blamed and reprimanded for a large financial error that is uncovered in the course of an external audit. Despite her protestations that the writing on the incriminating documents is not hers and that she was on a training course at the time it happened, her manager refuses to listen and says she will have to bring this matter to the attention of the senior accountant. Ms A goes home, and because she is so upset she visits her general practitioner the following day. He places her on sick leave for 3 weeks. He prescribes a hypnotic and anxiolytic to be taken as required. Just before the end of her sick leave her manager visits her at home to apologize, and admits her mistake. Ms A returns to work and her symptoms resolve over the subsequent week as she is welcomed back and made to feel appreciated.

Comment: If Ms A had responded to this stressful event with symptoms such as sleep disturbance, low mood, poor concentration, reduced appetite, and preoccupation at what had happened, she would be diagnosed with AD during the first 2 weeks with these symptoms, and if they persisted beyond that, she would then meet the criteria for depressive episode/major depression because the duration threshold would have been crossed. By the time her manager apologized, she might well be taking antidepressants and be labelled as having had major depression (DSM-5) or a depressive episode (ICD-10).

However, if she only had four symptoms in response to the event at work—such as sleep disturbance, low mood, impaired concentration, and reduced appetite—she would not reach the symptom number threshold at any time point, and even if the symptoms persisted beyond the usual cut-off for major depression, the diagnosis of AD would continue.

With the recognition of AD as a full-threshold disorder in ICD-11, she can be diagnosed with AD for the duration of these symptoms rather than the diagnosis changing once the 2-week threshold is crossed.

Initial controversies

Early criticisms

Since its inception, AD has provoked controversy on two fronts. The initial criticisms were concerned with the idea of identifying a new disorder for inclusion in the classifications. Some regarded it as essentially a 'wastebasket diagnosis' (16), assigned to those who failed to meet the criteria for other disorders, in order to ensure reimbursement for the treating doctors. So its inclusion in DSM-III was regarded as politically rather than scientifically motivated. Some argued that its validity was poor and that AD would mask prodromal schizophrenia, becoming the preferred diagnosis in adolescents. Linked to this was its diagnostic instability in this age-group, who, on readmission to hospital, often displayed symptoms of schizophrenia (17).

Others argued that the incorporation of AD constituted an attempt to medicalize problems of living, and did not conform to the criteria for traditional disorders such as having a specific symptom profile or psychobiology (18, 19). It was seen as a capitulation to a biological model, saying: 'as the progress of secularisation more and more reduces the medical to a purely biological, ubiquitous and socially inevitable, human adjustment problems are shunted away from a spiritual, moral and social form of accounting' (18). Despite these early criticisms, it has been retained in the further classifications, in large measure owing to its clinical utility, and AD now ranks as the seventh most frequently used diagnosis in a global sample of psychiatrists studied by the World Health Organization (WHO) (20).

The most substantial of these concerns related to the validity of AD, which has since been demonstrated. Among outpatients diagnosed with AD, there are differences from those given no diagnosis, but similarities on a number of parameters to those with depressive disorders; the diagnostic groups could also be distinguished by the type of stressor and the shorter duration of treatment in those with AD (21). Among medical inpatients (22), features distinguishing AD from major depression included age, marital status, symptom severity, and time to resolution of symptoms. Other studies demonstrating the predictive validity of AD confirm the good prognosis, with only 17%

developing a chronic course during a 5-year follow-up period (23) and a significantly lower 10-year readmission rate when compared to those with major depression (24).

In addition, quality of life was much less impaired in those with adjustment disorder than in those in other depressive disorder groups (25), while among self-harm patients (26), those with AD engaged in more impulsive acts—more often in association with alcohol abuse, and earlier in the course of the disorder, than those with major depression. They were also more emotionally deprived. Thus there are differences between AD and other depressive disorders on a number of parameters, and particularly in the predictive power of a diagnosis of AD.

More recently, mathematical models have been applied to demonstrate differences between AD and MDD (Casey and Shevlin, pers. comm.).

Later criticisms

A more recent strand of criticism has come from those who welcome the recognition that AD has afforded those experiencing pathological reactions—in response to stressors—that are frequently self-limiting, but nevertheless incapacitating. These critics question the approach of DSM-IV and -5 and ICD-10 to diagnostic criteria that are non-specific, and they also question the relegation of AD to secondary place in the diagnostic lexicon compared to other conditions (subthreshold status). They also argue that the approaches of DSM-IV and -5 and ICD-10 do not assist in resolving the boundary disputes that exist between AD and normal, adaptive stress reactions on the one hand, and between AD and major psychiatric disorders on the other (27, 28). These issues will be considered in detail in Chapter 3.

Why is AD important?

1. AD is a common diagnosis in certain clinical settings that include liaison psychiatry (29) and primary care (14). It is also the most common diagnosis made in those attending Emergency Departments following episodes of self-harm (30). Because of the frequency with which it is diagnosed, understanding its aetiology,

course, response to treatment, and prognosis is important so that those in whom the diagnosis is made can be provided with appropriate evidence-based treatments and receive accurate information on the likely outcome.

2. AD is also important as a differential diagnosis when other common mental illnesses are being considered. Because of the overlap with depressive episodes (DE) (major depression) and generalized anxiety disorder (GAD), these are often mistakenly diagnosed in preference to AD. This has implications for treatment as the interventions that are required for AD, if any, are likely to be brief and usually psychological rather than pharmacological, in contrast to those required for DE and GAD, which are often pharmacological, lengthier, and more complex (31).

3. A further concern relating to the accuracy of diagnosis is that one's self-perception is likely to be influenced by diagnosis. In particular, a person's own perspective on their life and their view of themself as having a potentially long-term illness, rather than a self-limiting stress disorder, are significant, and could potentially increase self-stigma and decrease self-esteem (32).

4. Service planning is based on, among other things, epidemiological evidence. The range of services for those with recurring illnesses such as DE is likely to be very different from those required to manage self-limiting conditions such as AD. Thus, the ability to clearly distinguish AD from other disorders in epidemiological studies which are the foundation for service development is crucial. If diagnoses are conflated and as a consequence a falsely high prevalence of one emerges at the expense of another, then there will be a mismatch between need and provision. This is particularly relevant if the disorder is self-limiting compared to that which is over-diagnosed and requiring various modalities of treatment and different forms of service delivery including stepped care. In this context, misdiagnosis or conflation of diagnoses will undermine service planning (33).

An example of the practical and personal implications of making a diagnosis of DE when a diagnosis of AD might be more appropriate is provided in Box 1.4.

Box 1.4 Case vignette 2: A potential false diagnosis of major depression

Ms A was a 66-year-old single woman, living with one of her sisters. About 20 years earlier she had been an inpatient in a psychiatric hospital for 3 weeks with a diagnosis of 'depression'. She took medication for a few months post-discharge and then discontinued them. Now, many years later, she took an impulsive overdose of aspirin because of a family feud about the ashes of her late sister. Prior to her death her sister was reported as not having expressed any wish regarding the dispersal of her ashes according to some members of her family who wanted to scatter them over her parent's grave, while others said she had expressed a wish to have them interred in her parents' grave. This difference caused a family dispute and Ms A, as the oldest sibling, tried to facilitate an agreement with both sides. She was frustrated when she was unable to achieve this. After the overdose, she was admitted to the psychiatric unit in the general hospital for observation. She was assessed by a doctor engaged in an antidepressant drug trial and permission was sought from the treating consultant to be included in this study. As the consultant was not certain that she had DE/major depression, permission was declined, pending further observation and assessment. Specifically, she had reported no mood changes until about 2 weeks previously when there had been a row with one of her siblings, to whom she had been very close, about the matter of the ashes. While an inpatient, she was reported as engaging well with staff, and her appetite was less than usual but there was no weight loss. She enjoyed friends visiting her and going out with them. She reported some concentration problems in terms of reading books, but was still able to read newspapers and watch some programmes on television. Sleep was diminished without hypnotics and she felt anxious, especially when the family were due to visit. She identified her low mood and anxiety as occurring largely when the family visited and the issue of the ashes was raised. She was adamant that the overdose had not been planned and she now regretted it. She described feeling frustrated at the protracted dispute despite her efforts to resolve it. After 2 weeks,

(continued)

Box 1.4 (Continued)

with support and encouragement from staff to distance herself from the dispute, her anxiety and appetite gradually improved and she was discharged home with community nurse follow-up and referral to the psychologist. She was also seen in the outpatient clinic over a 6-month period. Throughout this time, she was largely asymptomatic and the matter of the ashes was resolved between the siblings. A diagnosis of adjustment disorder was made.

Comment: Technically, this woman had DE/major depression because she reached the symptom number and duration threshold. Had this woman entered the drug trial she would have been viewed as having an illness that required an antidepressant for treatment, and a condition that might recur. She would have been subject to the rigors of repeated assessment and blood tests as part of a drug trial. A diagnosis of AD, however, indicates that the symptoms are driven by external factors and that when the person adapts to the stressor the symptoms will resolve, as they did in this particular case, after she had extricated herself from the role of mediator. The possibility that the symptoms on admission might represent a DE in evolution was considered but discounted when they improved over time and did not evolve further over a period of follow-up.

Conclusion

Since the first appearance of AD in DSM-III in 1980 (4), it has been a controversial diagnosis. The initial criticism stemmed from concern at the medicalization of problems of living, while the current controversies overlap since they are concerned with distinguishing between appropriate stress responses. Current opinion also goes beyond that and focuses on the distinctions between common mental disorders and the dangers of inaccurate diagnosis. The proposed ICD-11 (9) classification will further stimulate controversy and the extent to which the two classifications will diverge in their approach to AD. Even the most trenchant critics now agree that AD is an import diagnosis and that it warrants further research to secure its clear delineation from other diagnoses and to identify if, and when, interventions are required.

References

1. **Selye H.** A syndrome produced by diverse nocuous agents. Nature. 1936;**138**(3479):32.
2. **Levi L.** Society, stress and disease. Vol. 1: The psychosocial environment and psychosomatic disease. London: Oxford University Press; 1971.
3. **World Health Organization.** Mental disorders: Glossary and guide to their classification in accordance with the Ninth Revision of the International Classification of Diseases. Albany, NY: World Health Organization; 1978.
4. **American Psychiatric Association.** Diagnostic and statistical manual of mental disorders. 3rd ed. Washington, DC: American Psychiatric Association; 1980.
5. **American Psychiatric Association.** Diagnostic and statistical manual of mental disorders. 5th ed. Washington, DC: American Psychiatric Association; 2013.
6. **World Health Organization.** The ICD-10 classification of mental and behavioural disorders: Clinical descriptions and diagnostic guidelines. Geneva: World Health Organization; 1992.
7. **World Health Organization.** Mental disorders: Glossary and guide to their classification in accordance with the Seventh Revision of the International Classification of Diseases. Albany, NY: World Health Organization; 1955.
8. **World Health Organization.** Mental disorders: Glossary and guide to their classification in accordance with the Eighth Revision of the International Classification of Diseases. Albany, NY: World Health Organization; 1965.
9. **Maercker A, Brewin CR, Bryant RA, Cloitre M, Reed GM, van Ommeren M,** et al. Proposals for mental disorders specifically associated with stress in the International Classification of Diseases-11. Lancet. 2013;**381**(9878):1683–5.
10. **American Psychiatric Association.** Diagnostic and statistical manual of mental disorders. 1st ed. Washington, DC: American Psychiatric Association; 1952.
11. **American Psychiatric Association.** Diagnostic and statistical manual of mental disorders. 2nd ed. Washington, DC: American Psychiatric Association; 1968.
12. **American Psychiatric Association.** Diagnostic and statistical manual of mental disorders. 3rd ed. Washington, DC: American Psychiatric Association; 1980.
13. **American Psychiatric Association.** Diagnostic and statistical manual of mental disorders. 3rd ed (text revision). Washington, DC: American Psychiatric Association; 1987.
14. **American Psychiatric Association.** Diagnostic and statistical manual of mental disorders. 4th ed. Washington, DC: American Psychiatric Association; 1994.
15. **Zimmerman M, Martinez JH, Dalrymple K, Martinez JH, Chelminski I, Young D,** et al. Is the distinction between adjustment disorder with

depressed mood and adjustment disorder with mixed anxious and depressed mood valid? Ann Clin Psychiatry. 2013;**25**:257–65.

16. Fard F, Hudgens RW, Welner A. Undiagnosed psychiatric illness in adolescents: a prospective study. Arch Gen Psychiatry. 1979;**35**:279–81.

17. Greenberg WM, Rosenfeld D, Ortega E. Adjustment disorder as an admission diagnosis. Am J Psychiatry. 1995;**152**(3):459–61.

18. Fabrega H, Mezzich J. Adjustment disorder and psychiatric practice: cultural and historical aspects. Psychiatry. 1987;**50**:31–49.

19. Wakefield J. Diagnosing DSM-IV. Part 1: DSM-IV and the concept of disorder. Behav Res Ther. 1997;**35**(7):633–49.

20. Reed GM, Roberts MC, Keeley J, Hooppell C, Matsumoto C, Sharan P, et al. Mental health professionals' natural taxonomies of mental disorders: implications for the clinical utility of the ICD-11 and the DSM-5. J Clin Psychol. 2013;**69**(12):1191–212.

21. Despland JN, Monod L, Ferrero F. Clinical relevance of adjustment disorder in DSM-III-R and DSM-IV. Compr Psychiatry. 1995;**36**:454–60.

22. Snyder S, Strain JJ, Wolf D. Differentiating major depression from adjustment disorder with depressed mood in a medical setting. Gen Hosp Psychiatry. 1990;**12**:159–65.

23. Bronish T. Adjustment reactions: a long-term prospective study and retrospective follow-up study of former patients in a crisis intervention ward. Acta Psychiatr Scand. 1991;**84**:86–93.

24. Jones R, Yates WR, Zhou MH. Readmission rates for adjustment disorders: comparison with other mood disorders. J Affect Disord. 2001;**71**(1):199–203.

25. Looney JG, Gunderson EKE. Transient situational disturbances: course and outcome. Am J Psychiatry. 1978;**135**:660–3.

26. Polyakova I, Knobler HY, Ambrumova A, Lerner V. Characteristics of suicidal attempts in major depression versus adjustment reactions. J Affect Disord. 1998;**47**(1–3):159–67.

27. Casey P, Dowrick C, Wilkinson G. Adjustment disorders: fault line in the psychiatric glossary. Br J Psychiatry. 2001;**179**:479–81.

28. Baumeister H, Maercker A, Casey P. Adjustment disorders with depressed mood: a critique of its DSM-IV and ICD-10 conceptualization and recommendations for the future. Psychopathology. 2009;**42**:139–47.

29. Mitchell AJ, Chan M, Bhatti H, Halton M, Grassi L, Johansen C, et al. Prevalence of depression, anxiety, and adjustment disorder in oncological, haematological, and palliative-care settings: a meta-analysis of 94 interview-based studies. Lancet Oncol. 2011;**12**(2):160–74.

30. Taggart C, O'Grady J, Stevenson M, Hand E, McClelland R, Kelly C. Accuracy of diagnosis and routine psychiatric assessment in patients presenting to an accident and emergency department. Gen Hosp Psychiatry. 2006;**8**:330–5.

31. **Strain J, Friedman MJ.** Adjustment disorders. In: Gabbard GO, editor. Gabbard's treatment of psychiatric disorders. 5th ed. Arlington, VA: American Psychiatric Publishing; 2015. p. 519–29.

32. **Ben-Zeev D, Young MA** and **Corrigan PW.** DSM-V and the stigma of mental illness. J Ment Health. 2010;**19**(4):318–27.

33. **Regier DA, Kaelber CT, Rae DS, Farmer ME, Knauper B, Kessler RC,** et al. Limitations of diagnostic criteria and assessment instruments for mental disorders: implications for research and policy. Arch Gen Psychiatry. 1998; **55**:109–15.

Chapter 2

How common is adjustment disorder?

Patricia Casey

There are challenges to measuring the prevalence of AD in various populations. Despite the usefulness of the diagnosis of AD to psychiatrists (1), and even more so to psychologists (2), it has received little attention in epidemiological research. The most fundamental barrier is that there are no specific symptom criteria, and the only guide to making the diagnosis is the presence of a stressor and the subtypes (see also Chapter 1, pp. 3–4, Box 1.1). Some subtypes of adjustment disorder are difficult to distinguish from each other (3) as they are diagnosed on the basis of major features such as depression, anxiety, behavioural disturbance, or combinations of these.

A further problem in epidemiological research into AD is that it cannot be diagnosed once the duration or symptom threshold for another disorder is reached; this takes precedence over AD. This is known as the threshold problem. An example is provided in Box 1.3.

Additional difficulties exist regarding epidemiological studies of AD owing to the poor delineation of AD in the current diagnostic schedules, discussed below.

Diagnostic instruments—general

Most of the structured interviews do not include AD, probably owing to the absence of clear diagnostic criteria, unlike other disorders delineated in ICD-10 (4) and DSM-5 (5). Those not incorporating AD include the Clinical Interview Schedule (CIS) (6) and the Composite International Diagnostic Interview (CIDI) (7, 8).

By contrast, the Schedule for Clinical Assessment in Neuropsychiatry (SCAN) (9) and the Structured Clinical Interview for DSM-IV (SCID)

(10) include AD, but unsatisfactorily. In SCAN, the assessment of AD is located in Section 13, which deals with inferences and attributions. This comes after the criteria for all other disorders have been completed, and no specific questions are included to evaluate AD. Moreover, SCAN provides no guidance on the application of this section. By placing this near the end of the schedule there is a suggestion that AD is an unlikely diagnostic candidate for diagnosis. In SCID, the instructions to interviewers specify, as in ICD-10, that this diagnosis cannot be made if the criteria for any other psychiatric disorder are met since it is a subthreshold diagnosis. The Mini International Neuropsychiatric Interview (M.I.N.I.) (11) also incorporates a section on adjustment disorder but, as in SCID, AD is superseded when any another diagnosis farther up the hierarchy is made.

SCID (10) does include AD, but only if the criteria for another condition are not met.

Instruments specific to AD

Screening

Maercker and colleagues (12) suggest that, as with post-traumatic stress disorder, certain symptoms may define AD. These are intrusive symptoms/ruminations associated with involuntary stressful reminders, avoidance behaviour, and failure to adapt. The Adjustment Disorder—New Module questionnaire (ADNM) is the first screening instrument for AD based on these criteria. It allows for categorical and dimensional screening for suspected AD based on the new criteria (13, 14). The self-rated questionnaire is available in two versions, with either 20 items (15) or 29 items (13) in the form of statements covering intrusions, avoidance, failure to adapt, anxiety, depression, and poor impulse control. This symptom pool was derived from a survey of 22 experienced therapists in clinical practice. Each question is self-rated on the following parameters: acute/chronic, severity, and frequency. In addition, a list of stressors—seven acute and nine chronic—are presented which the individual 'ticks' as present or absent in the previous year and identifies the most prominent. This forms the basis for answering the symptom-related statements, the frequency of their occurrence, and their severity (one-off/acute, chronic, sporadic).

The 29-item ADNM (13) was validated on one group of patients with cardiac arrhythmias and on another attending a psychosomatic outpatient clinic. The factor analysis confirmed the three postulated symptom groups: intrusions, avoidance, and failure to adapt. The internal consistencies for these three scales ranged between 0.74 and 0.91. The test-retest reliability of the scales for a 6-week period lay between 0.61 and 0.84 and were acceptable except for certain types of coping strategies.

The 20-item scale was validated on a sample of burglary victims in Switzerland (15). The internal consistency was 0.94 for the total scale and 0.85–0.92 for the subscales. Test-retest reliability lay between 0.85 and 0.92. Further work on this scale (14) using latent class analysis and factor analysis identified six overlapping factors which the authors say represent a unifaceted concept of AD, and three latent classes representing severity. In essence, this means that no subtypes are recognized. A more recent study, also using a 20-item questionnaire, in a group of Lithuanian participants who had experienced at least one stressor in the previous year, found that a two-factor model was the best fit for the data—representing preoccupations and failure to adapt (16).

A 20-item version has been used in several studies (17, 18, 19), but at this point not more widely than by the researchers associated with the development of the new concept of AD for ICD-11. One of the reasons for this is likely to be that the proposed descriptor for AD has not yet been accepted for ICD-11. Another is that it may have limited generalizability owing to the specificity of the proposed criteria, particularly as they closely resemble those in post-traumatic stress disorder (PTSD) and the use of the ADNM might eliminate many of the patients currently diagnosed with AD using the broader ICD-10 and DSM-5 criteria.

One recent study in the *grey* literature, from Estonia (20), independent of the ADNM developers, found that among a group of subjects with possible AD only 6.5% were so diagnosed using the ADNM, while 80.6% were diagnosed clinically with AD. Construct validity was found to be poor. This may be explained by problems with the new concept of AD, with the ADNM itself, or by cultural differences in the study population compared to those in whom it was developed.

The development of another diagnostic instrument—the Diagnostic Interview for Adjustment Disorder (DIAD) (21)—was based on the DSM-IV definition of AD, but accords it full-syndrome status. The study sample was a group of people with disability diagnosed with or without AD using an algorithm using the DIAD. This 29-item schedule covers the stressors (items 1–3), then their onset and duration (items 4–6). Distress is evaluated (items 7–22), as is its onset (item 23). Next, the relationship between the distress and the stressor is evaluated (item 24), and finally the level of impairment (items 25–29). Both the content validity, using expert agreement, and the construct validity—compared against other measures of disability and distress—were satisfactory. Based on this schedule, Cornelius et al. (21) found a prevalence of AD of 7.4%, a much higher figure than that in other studies. Clearly, the emergence of this new schedule to facilitate a diagnosis of AD is welcome, although this study is the first effort at validation and further studies are required. It remains to be seen how well it performs in such studies.

Implications

Because of the inadequacy and scarcity of diagnostic tools there are few reliable studies regarding the epidemiology of AD, and so the current figures may not stand up to future attempts at replication. This is particularly true if the new concept of AD that has been incorporated into the ADNM is adopted in the future. A number of questions remain with regard to the new and old concepts of AD, and how these relate to its epidemiology. These are as follows:

1. Will the proposed definition identify the same group as those currently diagnosed with AD using the ICD-10 classification?
2. Will the new concept of AD be sufficiently distinct from PTSD, with symptom descriptions that emphasize the similarity of the two disorders?
3. Will ICD-11 adequately separate AD from normal reactions?
4. Will ICD-11 adequately separate AD from major depressive disorder or generalized anxiety disorder?

In respect of the second question, one field study using vignettes suggested that the psychiatrists were able to distinguish AD from

PTSD (22), although this may change when tested in clinical practice. There are no answers to the remaining three questions raised above.

Epidemiology

In this section, studies using the old and the proposed new concepts will be highlighted, although the latter are scarce.

A general concern is that the data on the epidemiology of AD should be treated with caution since the diagnosis is made by measures that are imperfect and that relegate AD to a subthreshold status. The impact of this is that reaching this threshold for another overlapping disorder leads to a diagnostic change—from AD, usually to major depression or generalized anxiety. The strict application of the DSM-5 criteria (5), and to a lesser extent those of ICD-10 (since it allows greater clinical latitude) (4), causes this artificial shift in diagnosis even when AD might be more clinically appropriate. Thus, most of these studies are likely to under-estimate its prevalence as AD may have had to be replaced by another diagnosis.

General population studies

None of the major international studies—such as the Epidemiologic Catchment Area (ECA) Survey (23), the National Comorbidity Survey (24), the National Comorbidity Replication Survey (25), or the National Psychiatric Morbidity Survey (26)—included AD among the conditions examined because the schedules used did not include AD. The first to do so was a multicentre study covering five European countries (27). It identified a prevalence of 0.5%, which varied across countries from 0 to 1.1 per 100,000. It was more commonly diagnosed in women than in men. This study used the SCAN interview, which does include AD but only after all other threshold disorders have been considered. It relegates AD to a left-over non-specific group.

Studies using the new concept of AD in the general population

As described above, ICD-11 proposes specific symptom criteria for AD (see also Chapter 1, pp. 7–8) that require preoccupation with the stressor and failure to adapt. Two studies have applied a version of the new criteria to a diagnosis of AD. Based on these criteria, a general population study (17) identified a prevalence of 0.9–1.4%, dependent on whether or not functional impairment was required, with a lower figure when functional impairment was required. It also found that in 72% of those with this diagnosis, symptoms had been present for between 6 and 24 months at the time of assessment, demonstrating that, in some, it is a long-standing condition. The triggers were acute stressors such as moving house, or chronic stressors; physical illness or conflict at work or with neighbours were the most common triggers. The importance of examining prevalence data with and without the impairment criterion is that the current ICD-10 criteria require both symptoms and impairment, while DSM-5 criteria require one or the other. The aforementioned figures show that there is likely to be a substantial difference in the number of cases diagnosed when both are required since the addition of impairment raises the threshold for diagnosis, resulting in a lower prevalence figure.

The second study to utilize a version of the proposed new criteria was conducted on those aged over 65 years (18). It found the prevalence of AD to be 2.3%, and the prevalence of major depression to be similar. In both of these studies the symptoms that constituted AD were avoidance, intrusions, and failure to adapt; however, avoidance has now been removed from the proposed new criteria and this might impact on prevalence data in future studies, making them higher than the above studies are indicating. It is arguable that the three symptoms proposed were too specific and would have aligned AD too closely with PTSD, thereby conflating the two and replicating the overlap with depressive episode and generalized anxiety (28); this has yet to be demonstrated empirically.

Even for those individuals exposed to severe events that are not directly life-threatening—for example, lack of shelter, loss of property, and hunger—some may develop AD and not PTSD. A secondary analysis (29) of a study of refugees used questions derived from other interview schedules measuring extreme stress. These included the core symptoms that were being proposed for AD in ICD-11 (intrusions, avoidance, and failure to adapt). A prevalence for AD of 5.7% (Ethiopia), 40.3% (Algeria), 16.1% (Gaza), and 30.7% (Cambodia) was reported (19), while the prevalence of PTSD was 15.8%, 37.4%, 17.8%, and 28.4%, respectively (29). There was high comorbidity between AD and PTSD ranging from 52.99% to 70.3% (19). This is hardly surprising given the commonality of the proposed symptoms for AD and those of PTSD.

General practice

The epidemiology of AD has been studied less frequently in primary care than other conditions such as major depression or generalized anxiety. Yet it is assumed that AD is more common in this population (30). One such study identified a prevalence of AD in 1% of consulters with mental health problems (31) using a clinical diagnosis based on ICD-9.

One study focusing on the anxious subtype of AD, and using the M.I.N.I. (11) to make the diagnosis, found that it was present in 1% of the total consulting population and in 4.5% of those with mental health problems (32). It used as its base 78 general practitioners from various regions in France. A further study involving 77 medical centres with 618 GPs in the Catalan region of Spain (33) found that the prevalence of AD was 2.9% when assessed using SCID. There was very poor recognition by the GPs, with only two out of 110 cases of AD identified by them. This is entirely predictable since the second edition of the WHO *International Classification of Primary Care* (ICPC-2) makes no reference to adjustment disorders (34). This study also found that of the subtypes, AD was more commonly diagnosed in the anxious group than in the depressive group, and also that AD was diagnosed less frequently than was either major depressive disorder or generalized anxiety. This was a surprising finding since it has been suggested that it is one of the most common disorders in primary care.

Psychiatric clinics

One of the first epidemiological studies of AD (35) observed that 5% of inpatient and outpatient cohorts were diagnosed with AD, while another (36) noted that 2.3% of those attending a walk-in clinic (a diagnostic and evaluation centre) met criteria for AD, with no other psychiatric diagnoses. When patients with other co-occurring psychiatric diagnoses were included, 20% had the diagnosis of AD.

A study of intake diagnoses in outpatient clinics, combining clinical evaluation and a structured interview using SCID, found that AD was the most common clinical diagnosis, made in 36% of patients, as compared to just over 11% using SCID (37). Among psychiatric inpatients, 9% of consecutive admissions to an acute public sector unit were diagnosed with AD (38).

Consultation-liaison psychiatry

Consultation-liaison (CL) psychiatry is the setting in which AD is most commonly diagnosed. A prevalence of between 11.5% and 21.5% has been identified by several investigators (39–41) in the general CL population, and AD is more common than is major depression or anxiety disorders (42).

Turning to specific groups, one study (43) identified 50% of cancer patients as having a psychiatric disorder, most commonly AD with depression, while another (44) identified AD in 27% and major depression in 23%. A more recent study (45), using a structured interview, identified a 4-week prevalence of 31.8% for any mental disorder, of which 11.1% had an AD while the remainder were diagnosed with any anxiety disorder, mood disorder, somatoform or conversion disorder, or substance misuse. It also reported breast cancer and head and neck cancers as having the highest prevalence for any mental disorder (over 40%), while pancreatic, stomach, and oesophageal cancers had the lowest prevalence (ranging from 12.8% to 21.2%). Among cancer patients experiencing a recurrence, AD is diagnosed in up to one-third of patients (46).

In palliative care, one meta-analysis based on 24 studies identified AD in 15.4% of subjects, in comparison to a pooled prevalence of 14.3% for DSM-defined major depression and 16.5% for either DSM- or ICD-10-defined depressive disorder (47). One concern about the diagnosis of AD in cancer patients in particular is the likely overlap with understandable distress, and the extent to which this was considered by those conducting these studies. Thus, while the prevalence of AD seems high in this group, it may be inflated.

Another study (48) examined the consultation-liaison psychiatric data from seven university teaching hospitals in the United States, Canada, and Australia, all of which used a common computerized database. AD was diagnosed in 12.0% of patients, was the sole diagnosis in 7.8%, and was comorbid with other psychiatric diagnoses in 4.2%. It applied a 'rule-out' diagnosis to an additional 10.6%. Comorbidity most frequently was with personality disorder and organic mental disorder. In their socio-demographic profiles, those with AD had less previous psychiatric illness and pre-morbidly were rated as functioning better than those patients with major mental disorders. All of these findings are consistent with the construct of AD as a maladaptive response to a stressor.

Among different age groups, one study (49) reported that 50.7% of patients aged 55 years or older who had had elective surgery for coronary artery disease developed AD from the stress of surgery, and in 30% it was still present 6 months after surgery. In a similar age group, Kellermann et al. (50) reported that 27% of elderly patients examined 5–9 days after a cerebrovascular accident fulfilled the criteria for AD.

Examining different medical and surgical diagnoses, AD was more commonly diagnosed than major depression in patients having head and neck surgery (13.1% vs 3.7%) (51), and the variables associated with either diagnosis after controlling for confounders were advanced stage of cancer and living alone. AD was also found in 73% of those with HIV infection (52).

Among patients with burns, a diagnosis of AD was made in over 60% of inpatient referrals, compared to less than 8% with either major depression or PTSD, and the severity or type of burn injury did not determine whether the diagnosis was PTSD or AD (53). This demonstrates that injuries that might be expected to cause PTSD do not necessarily do so, and so that PTSD is not inevitable. A study of victims of severe physical injury used structured interviews to evaluate the prevalence of AD (54), although a diagnosis was not made until 3 months post injury so as to exclude understandable distress. A prevalence of 18.9% was found at 3 months, and at 12 months one-third of these patients still met the criteria for the diagnosis while a further 20% had developed another unspecified diagnosis. Symptoms had resolved in the remaining 47%. New cases of AD emerged at the 12-month assessment, amounting to 16.3%.

Among those with neurological disease, AD was identified in 20% of patients in early stages of multiple sclerosis (55) and in 40% of post-stroke patients (56). A study examining the trajectory of mood changes following stroke (57) found that mood disorder post stroke

(MDPS) was present at day 5, at 1 month, and at 3 months in 5%, 16%, and 21% of patients, respectively. The authors speculated that 'early MDPS may reflect a more transient reaction or adjustment to the stroke, while late MDPS may reflect a neuroanatomical or neuropathological disorder related to the stroke that has a more delayed but enduring effect on mood'. Thus, AD is more likely present in the initial period, while major depression/depressive episode predominates in the later phase. Among dermatology patients admitted to a dermatology ward, 29% had a diagnosis of AD according to ICD-10 criteria compared to 34% having a depressive episode (58).

Despite the high prevalence of AD in a variety of consultation-liaison settings, the frequency with which AD is now diagnosed is declining, while the diagnosis of major depression is increasing (59). This may be due to real changes in the prevalence of AD, but a more likely explanation is that the availability of safer antidepressants over the past two decades, for those with medical illnesses, is impacting on and driving prescribing habits, ultimately impacting on diagnostic practice (59).

Emergency departments

The emergency department is the setting where most of all adjustment disorders are diagnosed. In one study, among those assessed in the emergency department following self-harm, a clinical diagnosis of AD was made in 31.8% of those interviewed, while major depression was less common at 19.5%. This pattern was reversed when a diagnosis was made using SCID (60). In another study (61), only using clinical diagnosis, 47.9% of those attempting suicide met the DSM-III-R criteria for AD, while 15.3% had other mood disorders. In the non-suicidal group, a diagnosis of AD was still more common (22.3%) than mood disorder (12.4%). Moreover, in those with AD the use of compulsory referrals to inpatient treatment was significantly higher when the reason for presentation was deliberate self-harm rather than some other event (46.7% vs 26.2).

Examining the totality of patients presenting to the emergency department, only paranoid schizophrenia (14.2%) and suicidal behaviours (12.1%) surpassed AD (6.7%) among those referred for psychiatric evaluation (62) based on retrospective evaluation.

Conclusion

The prevalence of AD varies with the population under study. It is highest in liaison-psychiatry settings and in patients seen in the emergency department. Studies in primary care have not found the high prevalence suggested by DSM-5, but that may be related to its under-recognition by general practitioners and to the unsatisfactory nature of the measures. The inclusion of AD in the category of Trauma and Stress-related Disorders in DSM-5 (5) is to be welcomed as this may bolster research in this area (63). The more recent tools developed may improve the detection and measurement of AD in a variety of settings. The use of the ADNM—based on a new theory of AD as a stressor-related disorder with a specific constellation of symptoms, overlapping with those of PTSD—may make comparison with earlier studies difficult. This requires further evaluation and represents an area ripe for further study.

References

1. Reed GM, Roberts MC, Keeley J, Hooppell C, Matsumoto C, Sharan P, et al. Mental health professionals' natural taxonomies of mental disorders: implications for the clinical utility of the ICD-11 and the DSM-5. J Clin Psychol. 2013;69(12):1191–212.

2. Evans SC, Reed GM, Roberts MC, Esparza P, Watts AD, Correia JM, et al. Psychologists' perspectives on the diagnostic classification of mental disorders: results from the WHO-IUPsyS Global Survey. Int J Psychol. 2013;48(3):177–93.

3. Zimmerman M, Martinez JH, Dalrymple K, Martinez JH, Chelminski I, Young D. Is the distinction between adjustment disorder with depressed mood and adjustment disorder with mixed anxious and depressed mood valid? Ann Clin Psychiatry. 2013;25(4):257–65.

4. World Health Organization (WHO). The ICD-10 classification of mental and behavioral disorders: Clinical descriptions and diagnostic guidelines. Geneva: World Health Organization; 1992.

5. American Psychiatric Association (APA). Diagnostic and statistical manual of mental disorders. 5th ed, revised. Washington, DC: American Psychiatric Association; 2014.

6. Lewis G, Pelosi AJ, Araya R, Dunn G. Measuring psychiatric disorders in the community: a standardised assessment for use by lay interviewers. Psychol Med. 1992;22:465–86.

7. Robins L, Wing J, Wittchen HU, Helzer JE, Babor TF, Burke J, et al. The Composite International Diagnostic Interview. An epidemiological

instrument suitable for use in conjunction with different diagnostic systems and in different cultures. Arch Gen Psychiatry. 1988;45(12):1069–77.

8. **Kessler RC, Ustun TB.** The World Mental Health (WMH) survey initiative version of the World Health Organization (WHO) Composite International Diagnostic Interview (CIDI). Int J Methods Psychiatr Res. 2004;13:93–121.

9. **Wing JK, Babor T, Brugha T, Burke J, Cooper JE, Giel R, et al.** SCAN. Schedules for clinical assessment in neuropsychiatry. Arch Gen Psychiatry. 1990;47:589–93.

10. **First MB, Spitzer RL, Gibbon M, Williams JW, et al.** Structured Clinical Interview for DSM-IV-TR axis 1 disorders, Research Version, Patient Ed (SCID-1/P). New York Biometric Research Department, New York State Psychiatric Institute, USA, Nov. 2002.

11. **Sheehan D, Lecrubier Y, Sheehan KH, Amorim P, Janavs J, Weiller E, et al.** The Mini-International Neuropsychiatric Interview (M.I.N.I.): the development and validation of a structured diagnostic psychiatric interview for DSM-IV and ICD-10. J Clin Psychiatry. 1998;59(S20):22–33.

12. **Maercker A, Einsle F, Kollner V.** Adjustment disorders as stress response syndromes: a new diagnostic concept and its exploration in a medical sample. Psychopathology. 2007;40(3):135–46.

13. **Einsle F, Kollner V, Bly S, Maercker A.** Development and validation of a questionnaire for the screening of adjustment disorder (ADNM). Psychol Health Med. 2010;15(5):584–95.

14. **Glaesmer H, Romppel M, Brähler E, Hinz A, Maercker A.** Adjustment disorder as proposed for ICD-11: dimensionality and symptom differentiation. Psychiatry Res. 2015;229(3):940–8.

15. **Lorenz L.** Adjustment Disorder New Module 20—construct validity, reliability and cut-off scores [Master's thesis]. Switzerland: University of Zurich, Institute of Psychology; 2016.

16. **Zelviene P, Kazlauskas E, Eimontas J, Maercker A.** Adjustment disorder: empirical study of a new diagnostic concept for ICD-11 in the general population in Lithuania. Eur Psychiatry. 2017;40:20–25.

17. **Maercker A, Forstmeier S, Pielmaier L, Spangenberg L, Brähler E, Glaesmer H.** Adjustment disorders: prevalence in a representative nationwide survey in Germany. Soc Psychiatry Psychiatr Epidemiol. 2012;47:1745–52.

18. **Maercker A, Forstmeier S, Enzler A, Krüsi G, Hörler E, Maier C, et al.** Adjustment disorder, post-traumatic stress disorder, and depressive disorders in old age: findings from a community survey. Compr Psychiatry. 2008;49(2):113–20.

19. **Dobricki M, Komproe IH, de Jong JTVM, Maercker A.** Adjustment disorders after severe life-events in four post-conflict settings. Soc Psychiatry Psychiatr Epidemiol. 2010;45(1):39–46.

20. **Viljus S.** Adjustment disorder new module: the adaptation and validation of a self-report questionnaire for the assessment of adjustment disorder [Master's

thesis]. Estonia: University of Tartu, Faculty of Social Science and Education, Institute of Psychology; 2013.

21. **Cornelius LR, Brouwer S, de Boer MR, Groothoff JW, van der Klink JJ.** Development and validation of the Diagnostic Interview Adjustment Disorder (DIAD). Int J Methods Psychiatr Res. 2014;**23**(2):192–207.

22. **Keeley JW, Reed GM, Roberts MC, Evans SC, Robles R, Matsumoto C.** Disorders specifically associated with stress: a case-controlled field study for ICD-11 mental and behavioural disorders. Int J Clin Health Psychol. 2016;**16**(2):109–27.

23. **Myers JK, Weissman MM, Dischler GL, Holzer CE 3rd, Leaf PJ, Orvaschel H, et al.** Six-month prevalence of psychiatric disorders in three communities 1980 to1982. Arch Gen Psychiatry. 1984;**41**:959–67.

24. **Kessler RC, McGonagle KA, Zhao S, Nelson CB, Hughes M, Eshleman S, et al.** Lifetime and 12-month prevalence of DSM-III R psychiatric disorders in the United States: results from the National Comorbidity Survey. Arch Gen Psychiatry. 1994;**51**:8–19.

25. **Kessler RC, Chiu WT, Demler O, Merikangas KR, Walters EE.** Prevalence, severity, and comorbidity of 12-month DSM-IV disorders in the National Comorbidity Survey Replication. Arch Gen Psychiatry. 2005;**62**:617–27.

26. **Jenkins R, Lewis G, Bebbington P, Brugha T, Farrell M, Gill B, et al.** The National Psychiatric Morbidity Survey of Great Britain: initial findings from the household survey. Psychol Med. 1997;**27**:775–89.

27. **Ayuso-Mateos JL, Vazquez-Barquero JL, Dowrick C, Lehtinen V, Dalgard OS, Casey P, et al.** Depressive disorders in Europe: prevalence figures from the ODIN study. Br J Psychiatry. 2001;**179**:308–16.

28. **Casey P, Dowrick C, Wilkinson G.** Adjustment disorder: fault line in the psychiatric glossary. Br J Psychiatry. 2001;**179**:479–81.

29. **de Jong JT, Komproe IH, Van Ommeren M, El Masri M, Araya M, Khaled N, et al.** Lifetime events and posttraumatic stress disorder in 4 postconflict settings. JAMA. 2001;**286**(5):555–62.

30. **American Psychiatric Association** Diagnostic and statistical manual of mental disorders. 4th ed. Washington, DC: American Psychiatric Association; 1994.

31. **Casey PR, Dillon S, Tyrer, P.** The diagnostic status of patients with conspicuous psychiatric morbidity in primary care. Psychol Med. 1984;**14**:673–81.

32. **Semaan W, Hergueta T, Bloch J, Charpak Y, Duburcq A, Le Guern ME, et al.** Cross-sectional study of the prevalence of adjustment disorder with anxiety in general practice [in French]. Encephale. 2001;**27**:238–44.

33. **Fernández A, Mendive JM, Salvador-Carulla L, Rubio-Valera M, Luciano JV, Pinto-Meza A, et al.** Adjustment disorders in primary care: prevalence, recognition and use of services. Br J Psychiatry. 2012;**201**:137–42.

34. **World Health Organization.** International classification of primary care. 2nd ed (ICPC-2). Geneva: World Health Organization; 2003.

35. **Andreasen NC, Wasek P.** Adjustment disorders in adolescents and adults. Arch Gen Psychiatry. 1980;**37**:1166–70.

36. **Fabrega H Jr, Mezzich JE, Mezzich AC.** AD as a marginal or transitional illness category in DSM-III. Arch Gen Psychiatry. 1987;**44**:567–72.

37. **Shear KM, Greeno C, Kang J, Ludewig D, Frank E, Swartz HA, et al.** Diagnosis of non-psychotic patients in community clinics. Am J Psychiatry. 2000;**157**(4):581–7.

38. **Koran LM, Sheline Y, Imai K, Kelsey TG, Freedland KE, Mathews J, et al.** Medical disorders among patients admitted to a public sector psychiatric inpatient unit. Psychiatr Serv. 2002;**53**(12):1623–5.

39. **Popkin MK, Callies AL, Colon EA, Stiebel V.** Adjustment disorders in medically ill patients referred for consultation in a university hospital. Psychosomatics 1990;**31**:410–14.

40. **Foster P, Oxman T.** A descriptive study of adjustment disorder diagnoses in general hospital patients. Ir J Psychol Med. 1994;**11**:153–7.

41. **Snyder S, Strain JJ.** Differentiation of major depression and AD with depressed mood in the medical setting. Gen Hosp Psychiatry. 1989;**12**:159–65.

42. **Silverstone PH.** Prevalence of psychiatric disorders in medical inpatients. J Nerv Ment Dis. 1996;**184**:43–51.

43. **Spiegel, D, Bloom JR, Kramer HJC, Gottheil E.** Effect of psychosocial treatment on survival of patients with metastatic breast cancer. Lancet. 1989;**14**:888–91.

44. **Grassi L, Gritti P, Rigatelli M, Gala C.** Psychosocial problems secondary to cancer: an Italian multicenter survey of consultation-liaison psychiatry in oncology. Italian Consultation-Liaison Group. Eur J Cancer. 2000;**36**:579–85.

45. **Mehnert A, Brähler E, Faller H, Härter M.** Four-week prevalence of mental disorders in patients with cancer across major tumor entities. J Clin Oncol. 2014;**32**(31):3540–6.

46. **Okamura H, Watanabe T, Narabayashi M, Katsumata N, Ando M, Adachi I, et al.** Psychological distress following first recurrence of disease in patients with breast cancer: prevalence and risk factors. Breast Cancer Res Treat. 2002;**61**(2):131–7.

47. **Mitchell AJ, Chan M, Bhatti H, Halton M, Grassi L, Johansen C, et al.** Prevalence of depression, anxiety, and adjustment disorder in oncological, haematological, and palliative-care settings: a meta-analysis of 94 interview-based studies. Lancet Oncol. 2011;**12**(2):160–74.

48. **Strain JJ, Smith GC, Hammer JS, McKenzie DP, Blumenfield M, Muskin P, et al.** AD: a multisite study of its utilization and interventions in the consultation-liaison psychiatry setting. Gen Hosp Psychiatry. 1998;**20**:139–49.

49. **Oxman TE, Barrett JE, Freeman DH, Manheimer E.** Frequency and correlates of AD relates to cardiac surgery in older patients. Psychosomatics. 1994;**35**:557–68.

50. Kellermann M, Fekete I, Gesztelyi R, Csiba L, Kollár J, Sikula J, et al. Screening for depressive symptoms in the acute phase of stroke. Gen Hosp Psychiatry. 1999;21:116–21.

51. Kugaya A, Akechi T, Okuyama T, Nakano T, Mikami I, Okamura H, et al. Prevalence, predictive factors, and screening for psychological distress in patients with newly diagnosed head and neck cancers. Cancer. 2000;88:2817–23.

52. Pozzi G, Del Borgo C, Del Forna A, Genualdo A, Mannelli P, Fantoni M. Psychological discomfort and mental illness in patients with AIDS: implications for home care. AIDS Patient Care STDS. 1999;13:555–64.

53. Perez-Jimenez JP, Gomez-Bajo GJ, Lopez-Catillo JJ, Salvador-Robert M, Garcia Torres V. Psychiatric consultation and post-traumatic stress disorder in burned patients. Burns. 1994;20:532–6.

54. O'Donnell ML, Alkemade N, Creamer M, McFarlane AC, Silove D, Bryant RA, et al. A longitudinal study of adjustment disorder after trauma exposure. Am J Psychiatry. 2016;173(12):1231–8.

55. Sullivan MJ, Winshenker B, Mikail S. Screening for major depression in the early stages of multiple sclerosis. Can J Neurol Sci. 1995;22:228–31.

56. Shima S, Kitagawa Y, Kitamura T, Fujinawa A, Watanabe Y. Post stroke depression. Gen Hosp Psychiatry. 1994;16(4):286–9.

57. Townend BS, Whyte S, Desborough T, Crimmins D, Markus R, Levi C, et al. Longitudinal prevalence and determinants of early mood disorder poststroke. J Clin Neurosci. 2007;14(5):429–34.

58. Pulimood S, Rajagopalan B, Rajagopalan M, Jacob M, John JK. Psychiatric morbidity among dermatology inpatients. Natl Med J India. 1996;9:208–10.

59. Diefenbacher A, Strain JJ. Consultation-liaison psychiatry: stability and change over a 10-year period. Gen Hosp Psychiatry. 2002;24(4):249–56.

60. Taggart C, O'Grady J, Stevenson M, Hand E, McClelland R, Kelly C. Accuracy of diagnosis and routine psychiatric assessment in patients presenting to an accident and emergency department. Gen Hosp Psychiatry. 2006;8:330–5.

61. Schnyder U, Valach L. Suicide attempters in a psychiatric emergency room population. Gen Hosp Psychiatry. 1997;19:119–29.

62. Kropp S, Andreis C, te Wildt B, Sieberer M, Ziegenbein M, Huber TJ. Characteristics of psychiatric patients in the Accident and Emergency Department. Psychiatr Prax. 2007;34(2):72–5.

63. Strain JJ, Casey P, editors. Conceptual framework and controversies in adjustment disorders. In: Trauma- and stressor-related disorders: a handbook for clinicians. Washington, DC: American Psychiatric Publication; 2016. p. 37–58.

Chapter 3

The diagnostic quagmire: Philosophical issues

Patricia Casey

The conceptualization and classification of adjustment disorder (AD) are intimately bound up with the classification of depressive illness as outlined in the historical background below.

The fathers of psychiatry—Emil Kraepelin, Kurt Schneider, and Eugen Bleuler—were focused on so-called endogenous mental disorders such as schizophrenia, melancholia, mania, and dementia. These arose not in response to any external triggers, but were internal to the individual. The focus changed under the influence of Freud, who demonstrated that external factors such as childhood trauma could result in 'neurotic' phenomena. This was also the view of Karl Jaspers (1), a philosopher and psychiatrist, who recognized the direct role of stressful events in causing mental disorders. He called these 'psychogenic' reactions and identified a clear causal connection between the stressor and the onset, content, and course of the symptoms.

Turning to 'depression' specifically, Hill (2) viewed this as comprising several domains—that is, as a disease, a reaction, a normal emotion, an existential problem, and a 'psychobiological posture'. Melancholia was the quintessential manifestation of depression as a disease. He regarded it as a separate entity within the depressive constellation. He believed that the manner in which it affected the individual was qualitatively distinct from normality and that it was biological in origin. Moreover, depression as a 'reaction' was viewed by Hill as a paradigm of the adaptive reactions of the organism to intolerable situations, while as a psychobiological posture he regarded depression as a form of communication. Thus, the term depression subsumes multiple different depressive conditions, each of which may have their unique or overrepresented causes, differing pathologies, and differing intrinsic capacities to respond to differing treatments.

Taylor (3) also suggested three domains—diseases, illnesses, and predicaments. The disease element was associated with structural change to tissue (i.e. biological), and was the most important, according to him, because it determined treatment and was independent of the patient's account, arguably because of the visibility of some of the symptoms such as psychomotor retardation. He defined illness as an 'experience' which may or may not be caused by a disease, and predicaments as the 'complex of psychosocial ramifications, contacts, meanings, and ascriptions which bear upon the individual'.

Nonetheless, studies from both sides of the Atlantic showing that life stressors could also play a role in triggering the onset of depressive conditions, formerly thought to be 'endogenous' (4, 5), became persuasive. This culminated in a decision by the American Psychiatric Association (APA) (6) to jettison concepts such as 'reactive' and 'endogenous' depression and merge them into a single unitary disorder known as 'major depression' in DSM-III (*Diagnostic and Statistical Manual of Mental Disorders, Third Edition*). ICD-9 (International Classification of Diseases, Ninth Revision) followed suit with 'depressive episode'. The unitary model continues to dominate psychiatry, although there have been dissenting voices and these are becoming more vocal.

The growth of the anti-psychiatry movement in the 1950s was as a reaction to what was seen as pathologizing the day-to-day problems of living. But it is no longer this group who are voicing concerns about the current classification, but prominent mainstream psychiatrists.

For example, McHugh (7) proposed separating mental disorders into four 'clusters'. The first comprised 'brain diseases that directly disrupt the neural underpinnings of psychological faculties' and reflected structural or functional pathology. The second represented vulnerability to mental disorders because of the person's psychological make-up, with a personality-based disposition that responded with greater distress to stressors. The third category constituted those who 'adopt a behaviour that has become a relatively fixed way of life', and the fourth cluster comprised patients with 'distressing mental conditions provoked by events thwarting or endangering their hopes, commitments and aspirations', with grief as one example.

Parker & Paterson (8) describe the continuing difficulties in distinguishing 'clinical' from 'non-clinical' depression. They suggest a two-pronged approach and hypothesize that the disease model be applied to the severe melancholic or psychotic depressive states, and that a dimensional approach should be used to describe the other depressive states in which the differing contributions of personality and psychosocial stressors are incorporated without any natural boundary between them. In the latter group is AD, with its strong causal relationship to stressful events but also its distinction from normal adaptive reactions.

Kendler (9), a supporter of operational definitions and of DSM-5 generally, has recently identified the inadequacy of the description of major depression in DSM-5 and commented that an impoverished view of the psychopathology of that condition has affected our research, clinical work, and teaching in some undesirable ways. This, he believes, is because of the rigid application of the criteria set out in DSM-5.

The models proposed by Taylor (3), Hill (2), McHugh (7), and Parker & Paterson (8) are relevant to AD in respect of where this fits into the lexicon of depressed mood currently, and where in future classifications AD might be placed, since the conceptualization of even major depression/depressive episode allows for the prominent role of triggering stressors in some cases.

Returning to the current unitary approach to 'depression', the acceptance that stressors could trigger certain disorders, and in particular major depression, raised two questions:

1. How can we distinguish normal reactions to stressors from those that are pathological?
2. How can we distinguish one psychiatric disorder (e.g. major depression) from another (e.g. AD) if both have triggers?

Zones of rarity

Zones of rarity refer to the clear lines of demarcation—the natural boundaries—that exist between normal responses and those that are pathological on the one hand, and on the other those that distinguish the various psychiatric disorders from one another (10–12). This binary approach is deeply rooted in the disease model, where a named disease is either present or absent. Applied to psychiatry, post-traumatic stress disorder (PTSD) should differ from major depression or from generalized anxiety disorder, and each in turn should be distinct from normal distress. This is the approach used in general medicine, where various diseases are recognized and distinguished from others by their symptoms, aetiology, pathophysiology, course and prognosis, and the process involved in each of these domains is termed validation.

DSM-III (6) was based on a descriptive approach to classification, so as to improve reliability. Symptoms and their duration were enumerated, and the belief of its architects was that this would be the foundation for research into the various psychiatric syndromes by relating them to genetics, psychobiology, treatment, and so on, so that clear cleavages could be identified between the various disorders. It was also envisaged that clear lines of demarcation would distinguish those with and without mental illness. The objective of identifying a zone of rarity using various parameters has not been realized, and the descriptive approach remains the mainstay of psychiatric diagnosis.

The failure to identify clear biological or genetic characteristics, symptoms, or other markers was disappointing for those developing the DSM-5 classification (13). It was suggested that only those syndrome categories that had been validated based on key measures such as prognostic significance, evidence of psychobiological disruption, or prediction of response to treatment should have been included in the main text (14). It was also suggested that weakly validated conditions should be placed in the DSM-5 appendix, to represent categories requiring further research. This would allow the validated syndromes to be further explored for information on aetiology, treatment, and prognosis, while the validity of the others could be further researched to potentially achieve some of the goals of DSM-III (6). This did not happen.

The absence of zones of rarity makes the separation of AD from normal stress responses very difficult. Maj (15) has pointed to the need for descriptions of normal responses to major stressors to assist in making this distinction, and while this is possible for grief (13), for the responses to disasters, life transitions, and so on, the sheer volume and combination of events that befall humans are limitless, making the task impossible. Indeed the term 'normal' seems like an oxymoron in some circumstances. For example, what is the normal reaction to seeing your child die on the roadside following a hit-and-run accident? What is the appropriate reaction to being told you have a life-threatening illness? What is the normal response to learning that your daughter has emptied your bank account in order to buy illicit drugs?

The absence of clear boundaries spills over onto recognized psychiatric syndromes so that the symptoms of one condition are also often found in others, calling into question the validity of many of the syndromes conventionally regarded as discrete psychiatric disorders (12). For example, some of the symptoms of the mixed anxiety–depression category are also found in generalized anxiety disorder. The impact of this is that definitive diagnosis has become difficult. Major depression, for example, is not a single entity, as is commonly and simplistically believed, but can have different manifestations in different individuals and various responses to treatment (16). Adjustment disorder overlaps with major depression (17), and even in PTSD—ostensibly more clearly defined—there are over 600,000 symptom combinations, making it so heterogeneous that multiple individuals with the diagnosis can have totally different symptom constellations (18).

Are there qualitative differences between normal and pathological sadness?

In attempting to distinguish normality from pathology, it has been assumed that there are qualitative differences between normal and pathological sadness, and that this overall qualitative difference is greater than the total depressive symptom score, being is an inherent feature of the depressive condition (19). Such differences have been explored, and the most common description among those with depressive illness, as distinct from normal sadness, was the experience of lethargy and inability to do things, whether because of tiredness or an inability to summon up the effort to do so. Also identified was a feeling of being inhibited and an inability to envisage the future, a sense of detachment from the environment, and physical changes similar to those associated with a viral illness (20). Interestingly, a sense of detachment was one of the symptoms that Kendler (9) noted was not included in the DSM-5 criteria for major depression. Clarke & Kissane (21) found that those who are merely sad are able to experience pleasure when distracted from demoralizing thoughts and the person feels inhibited in action by not knowing what to do, in contrast to the person with depressive illness who has lost motivation and drive, and is unable to act even when an appropriate direction of action is known.

Because the boundaries of mental illness such as AD, major depression, and PTSD are so elastic, there is a possibility that psychiatric illness will become a universal feature of human existence when no disorder is in fact present. This is known as the false-positive problem.

The false-positive problem and the DSM response

DSM-III (6) attempted to set out the broad requirements for deciding what constituted a psychiatric disorder. It stated that the response 'must not merely be an expectable and culturally sanctioned response to a particular event, for example the death of a loved one'. But 'expectable' is subjective, often judged through the prism of somebody who themself has never been exposed to such an event. Many experiencing 'expectable distress' cope; for example, after financial ruin there is a sense of disappointment, demoralization, and distress, but most do not require professional mental health services and over time they adapt to their new circumstances. Others become overwrought, develop significant depressive symptoms, or try to take their lives. In instances such as these, wisdom and experience—the attributes of good clinical judgement—may be a better guide to distinguishing normal from abnormal stress responses than scientific knowledge alone (22). This recognition of the role of clinical judgement is acknowledged in DSM-5 in relation to loss and major depression, but this is viewed by others as too subjective and a 'step backwards' (9).

The importance of distinguishing normal stress reactions from those that are pathological is summarized in Box 3.1. Diagnosing disorder where none is present has significant ramifications for the individual and for health policy.

> **Box 3.1 Importance of distinguishing normal from pathological reactions**
>
> Medicalization of suffering by using of 'treatments' (psychological or pharmacological) when none are required
> Stigmatization stemming from a mental illness diagnosis
> Difficulties for those falsely labelled as seeking subsequent health insurance, mortgages, etc.
> Self-perception as ill
> Inflation of epidemiological data due to false positives
> Inaccurate service planning based on such data

In the absence of biological markers to assist in identifying psychiatric disorder, what is to be made of psychological symptoms when people describe them? Concerns about the possibility of false positives led the architects of DSM-III (6) to try and divine the parameters of what constitutes a psychiatric disorder. The debate in the APA focused on homosexuality and whether or not it was a psychiatric disorder. In response, Robert Spitzer recommended that for symptoms to amount to a disorder they had to cause clinically significant distress *or* cause functional impairment. Since homosexuality per se was not associated with distress or impairment, it could not be classified as a disorder.

This clinical significance criterion is still used today in DSM-5 (ICD-10 does not use this) and it is seen as a way of reducing the problem of diagnosing psychiatric disorder when none is present. This is particularly prescient in respect of AD, where the difference between a normal reaction and one that is pathological is crucial but difficult to evaluate in clinical practice. In ICD-10, disorders have to have both symptoms and impairment (invariably) and thus a higher threshold is set for diagnosing psychiatric disorders than in DSM-5.

On examining the problems associated with false-positive diagnoses listed in Box 3.1, possible inflation of epidemiological data may seem improbable, but this has been demonstrated empirically when data from the Epidemiological Catchment Area (ECA) and National Comorbidity Survey (NCS) was re-analyzed. The addition of the clinical significance criterion resulted in a reduction in the 1-year prevalence estimates for 'any disorder' of 17% in the ECA study and of 32% in the NCS (23). Despite having its imperfections and its critics (24), the clinical significance criterion has some merit in helping reduce the false-positive rate.

Some argue (10) that DSM-5 has weakened the distress-dysfunction criterion by stating, 'Mental Disorders are *usually* associated with significant distress or disability in social, occupational or other important activities'. In practice, it is difficult to imagine how a psychiatric disorder could be present without at least one or other of these features (i.e. distress or impairment) being present.

ICD-10 neither uses the clinical significance criterion nor rigidly specifies the duration of symptoms; instead it allows for clinical judgement in making a diagnostic decision. It does require dysfunction to be invariably present, as well as symptoms. This applies to the new concept of AD proposed for ICD-11 (25) (see also Chapter 1, pp. 7–8 for details of these symptoms). One study of the new concept of AD in a general population sample found a prevalence of 0.9–1.4% based on whether or not functional impairment was required; the lower figure was associated with the requirement for impairment in functioning (26). These results confirm that requiring functional impairment as well as symptoms reduces data inflation.

The problem of distinguishing normal reactions from pathological responses is illustrated in Box 3.2.

Polythetic and monothetic approaches to symptoms

At present, any combination of a number of symptoms can lead to a diagnosis of a particular condition; this is the approach of ICD-10 and DSM-5. As a result, individuals with a similar diagnosis such as depressive episode have different constellations of symptoms and bear little clinical resemblance to each other. This clinical heterogeneity has been referred to on p. 39 of this chapter. This is known as the polythetic approach, in that no one symptom is essential and no particular constellation is required as all the symptoms are ascribed equal weight in reaching the diagnosis. There is a danger of false-positive diagnoses using this approach to classification. This is to be distinguished from the homothetic approach, in which specific symptoms are essential

THE DIAGNOSTIC QUAGMIRE: PHILOSOPHICAL ISSUES | **43**

Box 3.2 Vignette 2: The diagnostic challenge

Mr X claimed to have been adversely affected by problems at work. He was in middle management and said he had been bullied by his manager. He attributed this to the fact that he was gay, and gave examples of being verbally humiliated and shouted at in front of his peers, although he said none of these referenced his sexual orientation. Nevertheless, he believed this was an undercurrent, as did some of his fellow workers. He said that as a result of the problems, he experienced initial insomnia, psychic symptoms of anxiety but no physical symptoms, some impairment in concentration because of his preoccupation with his predicament (although he was able to carry out his work), and irritability with his colleagues at how he was being treated. He continued to work although he found this difficult and dreaded going to work each day. His mood was low and he had to have time off every few weeks in the form of a long weekend. He worried constantly about his problems at work. His GP commenced him on an SSRI (selective serotonin reuptake inhibitor) antidepressant without any effect. However, he enjoyed the company of his family, playing golf with friends, and going on family trips. During these periods his symptoms dissipated but he was always aware that on return to work they would re-emerge. He obtained a severance package from work and his symptoms resolved, followed 2 months later by new employment.

DSM-5 perspective: This gentleman could be diagnosed with AD since the symptoms arose in a particular context and reduced significantly when he was away from the source of his problems. He would also meet the criteria for major depression as he reached the distress criterion and the symptom duration threshold and number if one adhered rigidly to DSM-5.

ICD-10 perspective: If the ICD-10 criteria were applied, the level of impairment required for an ICD-10 diagnosis may not have been reached even if the required symptoms were present. Thus the possibility that this was an understandable response to a stressful situation should be considered.

This vignette illustrates the problem of ignoring the primacy that good clinical judgement should take account of the context of the

(continued)

Box 3.2 (Continued)

symptoms rather than basing diagnosis on symptom thresholds alone. While his 'symptoms' reached clinical significance in that he consulted his GP, still the antidepressants he was prescribed were unhelpful. The environmental change of getting a severance package and a new position resulted in symptom resolution. His symptoms were therefore self-resolving. Thus the diagnosis could be AD, major depression, or a normal stress response, depending on the criteria used and the flexibility with which are applied.

to making the diagnosis (termed the classical approach to categorization). It generates very narrow diagnostic criteria and leads to a strong resemblance between individuals receiving this diagnosis. It also carries the possibility of false negatives. A hybrid method could weight some symptoms more than others while not making them sufficient in themselves to make a diagnosis, but this has yet to be tested in psychiatry.

Boundary disputes with other disorders

Major depression

While there is controversy concerning the separation of AD from normal adaptive reactions on the one hand as discussed above, on the other there is a further boundary dispute between AD and other common mental disorders. This section will focus on the latter distinction. To date, there have been no studies examining the difference between AD and generalized anxiety disorder.

In distinguishing AD from other psychiatric disorders such as major depressive disorder (MDD), there is little of assistance except by the duration of the symptoms (14 days or more for MDD) and symptom numbers. Part of the difficulty stems from the fact that AD was deliberately designed to be phenomenologically non-specific (27). Only alterations in mood, anxiety, or conduct (or combinations of these) which are associated with distress *and/or* dysfunction in excess of what would be culturally acceptable for the stressor involved are required. Further, all of these are subjective assessments with no objective guidelines as to when they can be counted as criteria. Once the symptom number/duration threshold is reached, the diagnosis changes to that condition, making AD a subthreshold condition even when this might be the most appropriate diagnosis clinically. For example, a middle-aged man presenting following the loss of his engineering business during the recession, who describes low mood, reduced energy level and appetite, sleep disturbance, and impaired concentration due to constantly thinking about his situation, for 12 days will be diagnosed with AD, but if the duration of his symptoms is 14 days or more, his diagnosis changes to MDD. While a diagnosis of AD may seem clinically appropriate even after the 14 days, the change to MDD is necessitated by the duration criterion for MDD and the subthreshold status of AD. In the proposed criteria for ICD-11 the diagnosis will remain AD since it will be a full-threshold diagnosis in that classification.

The absence of diagnostic criteria has been of concern, and some have argued that ICD-11 should include specific criteria so as to give AD the recognition that it deserves as a psychiatric disorder and in order to stimulate research in this under-researched area (28). This has now been accepted and will come to fruition if the proposed criteria are accepted in ICD-11 (25) (see also Chapter 1, pp. 7–8).

Attempts to separate MDD from AD based on symptoms have not been very fruitful (see also Chapter 6, pp. 86–8) and neither symptom severity nor social dysfunction nor personality assisted (17), although the sample size in that study was small and the failure to identify differences may represent a type II error. Severity of depressive symptoms was the only feature that distinguished AD from MDD in the study by Fernández et al. (29), and when those with severe depressive symptoms were excluded there were no sociodemographic or stressor-related differences (30). A latent class analysis is currently under way, comparing AD with depressive episode (P. Casey, pers. comm.), and some symptoms are emerging as possible discriminators.

It is possible that other parameters, such as the threshold at which suicidal behaviour occurs or the longitudinal course, including readmission rates, may be of some assistance (see also Chapter 8, pp. 118–9), while the possible role of biological measures as a tool in diagnosis will be discussed in Chapter 6.

Other subthreshold depressive disorders

DSM-5, like its predecessors, regards those who do not reach the threshold for a specific disorder as having a subthreshold condition, so such disorders continue to be regarded as mental health conditions. Various epithets have been applied to disorders that fall within the depressive spectrum, including minor depression, subclinical depression, sub-syndromal depression, sub-syndromal symptomatic depression, non-specific depressive symptoms, and minor depression. The heterogeneity of the terminology applied to these conditions was highlighted in a systematic review by Rodríguez et al. (31). Subthreshold depression was mostly defined as depressed mood or loss of interest and with less than the five symptoms required to make a full-threshold diagnosis of major depression. The presence of symptoms in the absence of significant impairment was another criterion. For *minor depression* the highest level of agreement across studies was for not more than four symptoms lasting at least 2 weeks. *Sub-syndromal symptomatic depression* was defined in most studies using the definition proposed by Judd et al. (32): 'any two or more simultaneous symptoms of depression, present for most or all of the time, at least two weeks in duration, associated with evidence of social dysfunction, occurring in individuals who do not meet criteria for diagnoses of minor depression, major depression, and/or dysthymia'. Some definitions specifically excluded depressed mood or anhedonia, while others did not, and the required minimum number of symptoms varied from two to five depending on the specific terminology. From this study it is clear that the nosology used is, at best, confusing.

Surprisingly, *mild depression* is not a subthreshold condition but refers to major depression in which few, if any, symptoms are in excess of those required to meet the threshold for diagnosis. Moderate depression and severe depression represent an increase in the distress or dysfunction criteria.

Since AD is a subthreshold condition, it follows that if the focus is on aetiology, a person with less than the required symptoms for MDD, following a stressful event, could simultaneously meet the criteria for AD and also for one of the many subthreshold depressive conditions. The possibility of a symptom constellation meeting the criteria for two different syndromes, each requiring potentially different interventions, is indicative of the confusion and limitations of the wholly descriptive approach to psychiatric diagnosis that is currently in use. This anomaly would be less likely with the adoption of the ICD-11 since there is a specific symptom constellation required for AD and as it is a full-threshold disorder.

The only study to examine the overlap between subthreshold depression and AD evaluated those with 'depressive disorder NOS' ('DD-NOS', the term used for subthreshold depression in DSM-IV), and compared the findings to those with AD with depressed mood. Using 3,400 subjects, this study (33) revealed that those with DD-NOS were significantly more often diagnosed with comorbid social phobia and personality disorder. In addition, they reported more anhedonia, increased appetite, increased sleep, and indecisiveness, whereas those with AD reported more weight loss, reduced appetite, and insomnia. There was no significant difference between the groups in overall level of severity of depression or impaired functioning. There was a slightly elevated risk of depressive disorder in the first-degree relatives of those with DD-NOS. There have been no further attempts to replicate this study using a wider array of features or more sophisticated statistical analysis.

The National Institute of Mental Health riposte

The National Institute of Mental Health (NIMH) in the United States, headed by Thomas Insel, has been stridently critical of both the ICD and the DSM in recent years, and it has formulated a model that represents a paradigm shift in the classification of mental disorders. These are called the research domain criteria (RDoC) (34). They represent a framework for the study of mental disorders and encompass many levels of information from self-report to neuroscience (see Table 3.1). The NIMH believes that symptom complexes cannot be identified through clinical description and instead tries to relate the behavioural functions of the brain to the neural systems that underpin these symptoms.

In the RDoC there are five domains, known as positive valence systems, negative valence systems, cognitive systems, systems for social processes, and arousal/regulatory systems. Within each domain there are several constructs; for example, the constructs around positive valence systems include initial responsiveness, long-term responsiveness, reward learning, and habit. Each construct is then evaluated on the knowledge relating to each, and these derive from molecular studies, genetic studies, self-reports, and so on. These seven areas are known as 'pillars'.

The ideal of achieving the analysis required by this complex approach is a long-term, and arguably daunting, project. It is also clear that the excessive preoccupation with phenomenology as the external manifestation of an internal pathological process or disorder is too narrow. Take the case of PTSD, for example, with its symptoms such as flashbacks, which are supposed to be pathognomonic. One study (35) demonstrated that most people meeting the criteria for PTSD had not, in fact, experienced a traumatic event, and that the core features of PTSD such as arousal, avoidance, and re-experiencing were more common after everyday events, such as the death of a relative, than after events that were traumatic. This supports the view that relying on phenomenology alone is misguided (36) and that the domain approach espoused by Insel is to be preferred, albeit in the long term. An example of how the RDoC apply to AD pillars is illustrated in Table 3.1.

In a provocative piece, Tyrer (36) writes that the criteria for AD should be reframed because the phenomenology of stress and trauma is insufficient for diagnosis, saying, 'It is a handmaiden for the clinician, not a signpost to understanding'. He also believes in the need for an independent measure of stress, probably a neurobiological one, that is uncontaminated by the nature of precipitating factors in the behavioural response. For Tyrer, the role of personality is crucial; he advocates that those with recurring symptoms, in response to minor stressors, should not be so diagnosed, as these features are encompassed by the personality disorder diagnosis.

A view on how the gap between the symptom-based approach of clinicians and the domains and pillars of the RDoC can be bridged has been suggested by Maj (37) and includes symptoms linked to descriptions of dimensions such as neuroticism and externalization/internalization. Maj also identified a number of caveats, including the fact that neural circuits are involved in all mental processes, that

Table 3.1 Applying the research domain criteria (RDoC) to AD

The seven pillars of the RDoC	Central elements of pillar	Relevance to adjustment disorders
Translational research perspective	Basic science in the driving force behind the classification	Of some relevance as there is abundant evidence of neurobiological and behavioural consequences of stress
Dimensional approach to classification	Need to accommodate the full range of normality and pathology	Adjustment disorders are a good exemplar of a condition that has been neglected as outside the range of mainstream psychopathology and yet which is highly relevant to personal distress and functioning
Reliable and valid measures of diagnosis	Need for measures that are not artificially diagnosis-specific and which cover the range of all pathology	Highly relevant in adjustment disorders. The 'stress disorders' need to be accommodated as a broad group with standard measurements for all
Broader design of research studies	Need to acknowledge that treatments are effective across a range of disorders and the important variables are rarely diagnostic ones	Acceptance that adjustment disorders should be studied together with other stress disorders and not regarded as a separate entity
Integration of behaviour and neural science	Neural science determines behaviour and this should never be forgotten	Probably of limited value in adjustment disorders
Concentration on core concepts	Acceptance that a large number of disorders in DSM and ICD have limited validity and sustainability	Stress concept is a core one that is amenable to this model
Flexibility in accommodating new concepts	Currently too much attention is being paid to a range of specific DSM disorders that interfere with the evaluation of new ideas that may be of much greater heuristic value	The concept of adjustment disorders could certainly benefit from this, but only if there was a new understanding of how stress-related disorders are generated

there are concerns relating to the test-retest reliability of laboratory information, and possible delays in ever achieving the goals of integrating phenotypes and biology. An even greater challenge may lie in conveying the unique lexicon of the RDoC to working clinicians and the new way of approaching classification that this entails.

Conclusion

Philosophers of science and medicine have always had an interest in mental illness, and its boundaries with respect to AD have been of particular interest. Yet, as with most psychiatric disorders, there is overlap, and there are no symptoms or other features that demarcate one disorder from another: these are called 'zones of rarity'. DSM distinguishes symptoms that indicate illness from those that are appropriate and adaptive using the clinical significance criterion. Some regard this as too vague and ICD does not refer to this concept. The multitude of symptoms that currently define all psychiatric disorders (the polythetic approach) has so many combinations of possible symptoms that many individuals could have the same diagnosis with no overlapping symptoms. It was envisaged that by the beginning of this millennium our understanding of the biological and genetic aspects of mental illness would have allowed those developing the new classifications to use these additional measures, alongside the traditional phenomenological descriptions of symptoms, to compile a more scientifically coherent classification that would overcome the problems mentioned above. This has not happened, and work on the RDoC, promoted by the NIMH, continues.

References

1. Jaspers K. 1913. Allgemeine Psychopathologie. Translated *General Psychopathology—Volumes 1 & 2*. Hoenig J and Hamilton MW (translators). Baltimore and London: Johns Hopkins University Press; 1997.
2. Hill D. Depression: disease, reaction, or posture? Am J Psychiatry. 1968;**125**:445–57.
3. Taylor D. The components of sickness: diseases, illnesses, and predicaments. Lancet. 1979;**314**:1008–10.
4. Kendell RE. The classification of depressions: a review of contemporary confusion. Br J Psychiatry. 1976;**129**:15–28.
5. Akiskal HS, McKinney WT. Overview of recent research in depression: integration of ten conceptual models into a comprehensive clinical frame. Arch Gen Psychiatry. 1975;**32**:285–305.

6. **American Psychiatric Association.** Diagnostic and statistical manual of mental disorders. 3rd ed. Washington, DC: American Psychiatric Association; 1980.

7. **McHugh PR.** Striving for coherence: psychiatry's efforts over classification. JAMA. 2005;**293**:2526–8.

8. **Parker G, Paterson A.** Differentiating 'clinical' and 'non-clinical' depression. Acta Psychiatr Scand. 2015;**131**(6):401–7.

9. **Kendler K.** Book review. The loss of sadness: how psychiatry transformed normal sorrow into depressive disorder, by Horwitz AV, Wakefield JC. Psychol Med. 2008;**38**:148–50.

10. **Cooper R.** Avoiding false positives: Zones of rarity, the threshold problem and the DSM clinical significance criterion. Can J Psychiatry. 2013; **58** (11). 606–11.

11. **Wakefield J.** Diagnosing DSM-IV- part 1: DSM-IV and the concept of disorder. Behav Res Ther. 1997; 35 (7): 633–49.

12. **Kendall R and Jablensky A.** Distinguishing between the validity and utility of psychiatric diagnoses. Am J Psychiatry. 2003; **160**: 2–12.

13. **American Psychiatric Association.** Diagnostic and statistical manual of mental disorders. 5th ed. Washington, DC: American Psychiatric Association; 2013.

14. **Stein DJ, Phillips KA, Bolton D, Fulford KW, Sadler JZ, Kendler KS.** What is a mental/psychiatric disorder? From DSM-IV to DSM-V. Psychol Med. 2010;**40**(11):1759–65.

15. **Maj M.** From 'madness' to 'mental health problems': reflections on the evolving target of psychiatry. World Psychiatry. 2012;**11**(3):137–8.

16. **Parker G.** How should mood disorders be modelled? Aust N Z J Psychiatry. 2008;**42**:841–50.

17. **Casey P, Maracy M, Kelly BD, Lehtinen V, Ayuso-Mateos J-L, Dalgard OS,** et al. Can adjustment disorder and depressive episode be distinguished? Results from ODIN. J Affect Disord. 2006;**92**(2–3):291–7.

18. **Galatzer-Levy IR, Bryant RA.** 636,120 ways to have posttraumatic stress disorder. Perspect Psychol Sci. 2013;**8**(6):651–62.

19. **Helmchen H, Linden M.** Subthreshold disorders in psychiatry: clinical reality, methodological artefact, and the double-threshold problem. Compr Psychiatry. 2000;**41**:1–7.

20. **Costello CG, Healy D.** Dysphoria. In: Costello CG, editor. Symptoms of depression. Wiley; 1993.

21. **Clarke DM, Kissane DW.** Demoralization: its phenomenology and importance. Aust N Z J Psychiatry. 2002;**36**:733–42.

22. **Maj M.** 'Clinical judgment' and the DSM-5 diagnosis of major depression. World Psychiatry. 2013;**12**(2):89–91.

23. **Narrow WE, Rae DS, Robins LN, Regier DA.** Revised prevalence estimates of mental disorders in the United States: using a clinical significance criterion to reconcile 2 surveys' estimates. Arch Gen Psychiatry. 2002;**59**(2):115–23.

24. **Frances A.** Problems in defining clinical significance in epidemiological studies. Arch Gen Psychiatry. 1998;**55**:119.

25. **Maercker A, Einsle F, Kollner V.** Adjustment disorders as stress response syndromes: a new diagnostic concept and its exploration in a medical sample. Psychopathology. 2007;**40**(3):135–46.

26. **Maercker A, Forstmeier S, Pielmaier L, Spangenberg L, Brähler E, Glaesmer H.** Adjustment disorders: prevalence in a representative nationwide survey in Germany. Soc Psychiatry Psychiatr Epidemiol 2012;**47**:1745–52.

27. **Strain JJ, Friedman MJ.** Considering adjustment disorders as stress response syndromes for DSM-5. Depress Anxiety 2011;**28**:818–23.

28. **Baumeister H, Maercker A, Casey P.** Adjustment disorder with depressed mood. Psychopathology. 2009;**42**(3):139–47.

29. **Fernández A1, Mendive JM, Salvador-Carulla L, Rubio-Valera M, Luciano JV, Pinto-Meza A, et al.** DASMAP investigators. Adjustment disorders in primary care: prevalence, recognition and use of services. 2012;**201**:137–42.

30. **Barnow S, Linden M, Lucht M, Freyberger HJ.** The importance of psycho-social factors, gender, and severity of depression in distinguishing between adjustment and depressive disorders. J Affect Disord. 2002;**72**(1):71–8.

31. **Rodríguez MR, Nuevo R, Chatterji S, Ayuso-Mateos JL.** Definitions and factors associated with subthreshold depressive conditions: a systematic review. BMC Psychiatry 2012;**12**:181.

32. **Judd LL, Rapaport MH, Paulus MP, Brown JL.** Subsyndromal symptomatic depression: a new mood disorder. J Clin Psychiatry. 1994;**55**(April suppl):18–28.

33. **Zimmerman M, Martinez JH, Dalrymple K, Chelminski I, Young D.** 'Subthreshold' depression: is the distinction between depressive disorder not otherwise specified and adjustment disorder valid? J Clin Psychiatry. 2013;**74**(5):470–6.

34. **Insel TR.** The NIMH Research Domain Criteria (RDoC) Project: precision medicine for psychiatry. Am J Psychiatry. 2014;**171**(4):395–97.

35. **Mol SSL, Arntz A, Metsemakers JFM, Dinant GJ, Vilters-van Montfort PA, Knottnerus JA.** Symptoms of post-traumatic stress disorder after non-traumatic events: evidence from an open population study. Br J Psychiatry. 2005;**186**:494–9.

36. **Tyrer P.** Limits to the phenomenological approach to the diagnosis of adjustment disorders. In: **Casey PR and Strain JJ** (editors). Trauma and stressor-related disorders: A handbook for clinicians. Arlington, VA: American Psychiatric Association; 2016.

37. **Maj M.** Narrowing the gap between ICD/DSM and RDoC constructs: possible steps and caveats. World Psychiatry. 2016;**15**(3):1913–14.

Chapter 4

Models, risks, and protections

Patricia Casey

Historically, AD is described in a broadly similar way in both the DSM (*Diagnostic and Statistical Manual of Mental Disorders*) and the ICD (International Classification of Diseases). The closest equivalents to AD in the seventh revision of the ICD (1) were the terms 'anxiety reaction NOS', one of the conditions in the category *Anxiety Reaction without Mention of Somatic Symptoms*, and 'reactive depression' and 'psychogenic depression' in the category *Neurotic-depressive Reaction*. ICD-8 (2) introduced the term 'transient situational disturbance' and changed it to 'adjustment reaction' with the publication of ICD-9 (3) and to 'adjustment disorder' in ICD-10 (4). In the clinical description of the condition it states that personal vulnerability plays a role. It is unclear whether this refers to personality or to some other aspects of vulnerability such as lack of social support. Adjustment disorder will continue to be the term used in ICD-11 (5), but there is no mention of personal vulnerability in the proposed description.

DSM-I (6) introduced the category of transient situational personality disorder, also suggesting personal vulnerability. This was refined to acute situational disorder in DSM-II (7) to encapsulate any transient reaction to overwhelming stress in an individual without any apparent underlying mental disorder, thus removing the concept of personal vulnerability. Although it was supposed not to be diagnosed when another major disorder was present, this dictum was often ignored.

DSM-III (8) changed to the new term 'adjustment disorder', and eliminated the lifespan terminologies, replacing them with subtypes based on the main mood and/or behavioural features. The subtypes included the depressive, the anxious, the mixed anxiety and depression, the disturbance of conduct, and the disturbance of conduct and emotions groups, and/or with work inhibition, withdrawal, and atypical features. The revision of DSM III-R in 1987 (9) made further modifications that included a specifier of 6 months' duration and a subtype 'with physical symptoms'. It also changed the requirement for psychosocial stressors to, simply, 'stressors'. This was based on the recognition that stressors other than those which were psychosocial could cause AD, such as major surgery or a nuclear disaster (e.g., Chernobyl). DSM-IV (10) removed some of the subtypes and added an acute and chronic specifier. In the DSM classification AD was an orphaned category, but DSM-5 (11) has included it in the Trauma and Stress-related Disorders grouping.

Apart from the possible role of personal vulnerability, jettisoned from DSM-II (7) but still retained in ICD-10 (4), there does not appear to have been consideration of any coherent model. AD is positioned in territory between normal responses to stress and major psychiatric disorder in which there is a known aetiological agent.

Some have suggested a more pragmatic reason for the term, claiming that AD was designed as a 'wild card' to allow the coding of a psychiatric 'diagnosis' for work done by psychiatrists and other mental healthcare specialists when the patient's symptoms do not reach the criterion of a major mental disorder. Thus it fulfilled the requirement of having a diagnosis and acceptable code for insurance reimbursement. For this reason, the criteria were kept vague (12).

The stress/trauma model

The approach adopted by ICD-2 is based on the model presented by Horowitz (13), which postulates that AD and post-traumatic stress disorder (PTSD) are located on a stress–response continuum. Several phases are postulated. The first includes emotions such as fear but is also associated with denial and a refusal to accept the implications of the event. The third phase is associated with sadness or anger, leading to a desire to avoid thoughts and reminders of the stressful event. This fluctuates between intrusions and suppression of unwanted thoughts. Fluctuating waves of emotion are present. Intrusive memories (i.e., preoccupations) develop as the stressful information is inconsistent with existing schemata and these are stored in active memory. The stress–response process is concluded by a working-through phase that results either in adapting to the implications of what had happened or in mental disorder or personality change (see Fig. 4.1).

This is very similar to the typical grief response described by, for example, Kübler-Ross (14). Although the empirical evidence for these consecutive phases is sparse (15), some (e.g. Maciejewski et al.) (16) support this model but with a different order to the stages.

The crisis model

While the origins of crisis theory are attributed to Lindemann (17), the work of Gerald Caplan (18) was seminal in developing a crisis model and understanding the necessary responses to this. Caplan's interest in crises resulted from his work with families immigrating to

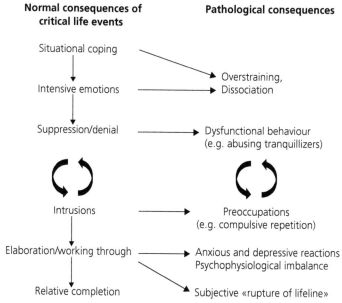

Fig. 4.1 Model of normal and pathological stress.
Reproduced from Psychother Psych Med, 61(3/04), Simmen-Janevska K, Maercker A; Anpassungsstörungen: Konzept, Diagnostik und Interventionsansätze [Adjustment Disorders: Model, Assessments and Interventions], pp. 183–192, Copyright (2011), with permission from Thieme Medical Publishers.

Israel following World War II. His model is based on the theory of homeostasis, in which the organism attempts to maintain a balance with the environment. In the initial phase the person responds to a threat to their homeostatic state with a rise in tension and attempts to quell it by drawing on their usual problem-solving methods. If this is not successful there is a further rise in tension and the feelings of threat continue, causing impaired functioning and feelings of distress. This further stimulates a rise in tension and the mobilization of emergency and novel problem-solving techniques. This may redefine the problem: the person may accept it or may find a solution. Finally, if no solution is identified, tension continues to rise and there may be a breakdown in the individual's social and mental functioning.

Caplan's (1964) crisis model (19) postulates typical trajectories that occur after stressful and destabilizing life events. The life event is considered a problem or demand that is currently unsolvable for the individual and results in a personal crisis. Insufficient or ineffective coping mechanisms result in psychological breakdown and stress-related mental disorders.

Another applicable model is the Lazarus & Folkman (20) cognitive-transactional model of stress. This model posits that individuals vary greatly in their appraisal of the stressfulness of any event. There are some stressors that everybody would regard as extremely stressful, and others that almost everybody would regard as mildly so. In this model an individual could achieve high stress scores from one or more very stressful events, or alternatively from a larger number of less stressful events, or even from a number of everyday events. Those who appraise minor stressors as very stressful may be innately or temporarily more vulnerable and less able to cope. Some may develop a disorder due to their vulnerability even when their total stress score is less than that in those without disorder. In general, the relationship between cumulative stressors and poor mental health is correlative, but modestly so (21). A study among 'depressed' college students (22) found that the level of stress per stressor, referred to as 'stress reactivity', was a better predictor of mental health problems than was the cumulative total stress score. Stress reactivity was also moderately correlated with neuroticism, thus compromising the person's coping skills. Since minor stressors abound and reactivity to these is a predictor of low mood, an intervention that focused on reducing reactivity might ameliorate the negative consequences of this. So, approaches to modifying the cognitive appraisal of these minor stressors, and approaches that influence the relationship between stress and their outcomes, are needed. These will be discussed further on p. 62, Vignette 3 of this chapter.

The biological model

While Caplan, like Horowitz, took an essentially psychoanalytic-therapeutic perspective, Selye (23) chose a biological approach that regards stress as a non-specific reaction to any kind of environmental demand, with symptoms increasing as the alloplastic load increases. This model highlighted the key role of the hypothalamic-pituitary-adrenocortical (HPA) axis in the human stress response. Pathological symptoms develop when there is an imbalance of arousal and inhibitory processes with altered HPA mechanisms (24), although there has been little research into the psychobiology of AD specifically.

Risk factors in AD

To date, the mechanisms underlying the development of AD have not yet been addressed sufficiently in AD research, though the ICD-10 particularly stresses the role of predisposition and individual vulnerability. In general, women are given the diagnosis of AD slightly more often than men (25). Overall, the risk factors seem little different from those identified for other common mental disorders. However, the studies prior to 2000 come with a health warning in that they did not control for confounders, thus rendering some of the results unreliable.

Life events and stressors

Adjustment disorder cannot be diagnosed unless there is a stressor in close temporal relationship to the onset of symptoms and which predates the emergence of symptoms. ICD-10 specifies the symptom emergence within 1 month, while DSM-5 specifies 3 months. Depressive episodes can also be triggered by a stressful event, but while this is not a requirement there is evidence that over 80% of episodes have such an antecedent for the index episode (26). In those with AD, as in PTSD, it is thus assumed that the disorder would not have arisen without this stressor.

It is unclear whether AD develops as the result of a single stressor in a vulnerable person, or cumulative stressors in a more resilient person. AD can occur with common events such as relationship breakdown or even with the type of events that lead to PTSD. In some instances, following a traumatic event, the full panoply of PTSD symptoms may be absent, and then AD is the more appropriate diagnosis. Comparing those with major depression in whom a stressful event had triggered the symptoms, with those diagnosed with AD, one study identified more events relating to marital problems and fewer of an occupational or familial nature in the AD group (26). This difference is unlikely to be of clinical utility since these stressors are non-specific.

Personality

Personality is assumed to be an important clinical factor for successful adjustment in stressful situations, and AD shows a comorbidity with personality disorder of between 15% and 73% (26, 27), but a recent study found that the comorbidity of possible personality disorder was significantly less for AD (56%) than for depressive episode (65%) (27). Thus, personality disorder is not a specific risk factor.

The personality dimensions of neuroticism, introversion, and psychoticism have been shown to be associated with heightened AD risk (28), as have the traits of harm-avoidance, and low scores on co-operativeness, self-directedness, and self-transcendence (29).

Coping

Neuroticism and introversion are related to maladaptive coping behaviours, such as the use of passive, self-blaming, and avoidant strategies to cope with stress (30, 31), which in turn have been connected to a higher symptom load in AD (32). Taking a dyadic perspective, one study found that the presence of depressive disorder in the female spouse increased the risk for AD symptoms among men of the general population, possibly due to the loss of dyadic coping strategies (33) Taken together, these studies indicate that maladaptive coping or poor support can be considered a risk factor in the development of AD.

Social and interpersonal factors

Patients suffering from AD have been shown to report significantly less social support than healthy controls (34). Alexithymia, or the limited ability to experience and describe emotions as conscious feelings, is considered a risk factor for AD also (35). Owing to poor social skills, it is likely that such individuals receive less social support in adverse situations. Reluctance to discuss a stressful event, and deficits in motivation regulation, were also shown to be associated with AD (36). It has been suggested that attachment style may be a risk factor for AD and that over-protectiveness may increase an individual's vulnerability to abnormal stress reactions; early separation anxiety in the individual may be the mediator (31, 37). Traumatic childhood experiences such as abuse have been shown to play a role in the severity of the disorder (37). The author of this study suggests that childhood trauma, over which the child has no control, results in a cognitive style of helplessness that causes distress and depressive symptoms.

Among those with AD who self-harm, emotional deprivation in childhood, a family history of psychiatric illness, or being from a one-parent-family or orphaned were significantly more common than in those with major depression who self-harm (38).

Indirect studies have not examined AD specifically but instead have examined conditions such as 'reactive depression', 'non-endogenous depression', or 'situational depression'. Thus there is a caveat attached to them. They are also old. Paykel et al. (39) found that the strongest relationship was between pre-morbid neuroticism and a non-endogenous symptom pattern with evidence of 'oral-dependent' personality. Findings linking neuroticism to a non-endogenous pattern of symptoms have been described by others (e.g. Benjaminsen) (40) in studies of subjects and their relatives (41).

Protective factors in AD—resilience

There is a clear need to better understand the psychobiology of resilience as an important element in the treatment of stress-induced dysfunction and distress (42), such as occurs in PTSD and AD. Much of the work on resilience has been carried out on soldiers and other combatants returning from war and by examining the attributes of those who develop adverse reactions such as PTSD. Holocaust survivors and victims of child abuse or those subjected to torture have also been studied. At community level, the 9/11 terrorist attacks in the United States provided much useful data also, and those exposed to natural disasters have been studied too.

There is little or no research on resilience in AD, but the questions that apply to any of the stressor-induced disorders such as PTSD are also applicable to AD. What are the attributes that result in one soldier becoming so overwrought that suicide is the outcome, while another, exposed to the same events, makes a successful return to family and community life? Why does one person react by self-harming when their marriage breaks down, while another, although upset, carries on, overcomes their sadness, and may feel that this event has given them positive insights? The focus in the past was on the psychological and social factors that enabled an adaptive response to stressors, but recently biological factors have also been considered.

Resilience is a process that facilitates the attainment of positive adaptation within the context of significant adversity. It can be described as 'bending but not breaking'. Resilience is not defined by the absence of symptoms but as marshalling certain coping skills that assist in maintaining equilibrium in the face of adversity. Faced with chronic stress, the person responds in a manner that results in positive adaptation.

Psychiatry has been focused on illness rather than resilience, and until recently resilience has been neglected by the specialty, in spite of the fact that it, rather than illness, is the most common response to adversity. Resilience is not static; an individual may be resilient to one stressor but not to another, and at one time of life but not another. There is no single pathway to resilience but rather multiple factors that contribute, some of which can be influenced and moulded, while others are fixed.

Among the characteristics of resilient individuals, the predominant ones are optimism, cognitive flexibility, active coping, social support networks, having a personal moral compass, and physical activity. A standardized, self-report assessment tool such as the Connor-Davidson Resilience Scale (CD-RISC) (43) can be of clinical assistance in identifying the areas of strength and weakness in a stressful situation. This may also enhance opportunities for intervention. It is an easy 25-item scale that is measured on a 5-point scale. Its psychometric properties are good.

While optimism is generally regarded as a fixed personality attribute, there is evidence that it fluctuates and assists in coping with severe illness and life transitions and in dealing with stressful events or traumas (44).

Cognitive flexibility refers to the ability to re-evaluate one's situation, as a consequence of new developments or simply as a result of change with the passage of time. Reappraisal can also involve finding meaning and positive outcomes, as well as acknowledging the negative and painful consequences. Stressful or traumatic events can be re-examined, altering the perceived value and importance of the event.

Active coping involves engaging in activities to achieve an outcome in response to the stressor. The opposite is passively waiting for a result. Active copers are mindful that they may become consumed by the stressor and they positively engage with others who can assist and support them. Instead of attempting to bring about a satisfactory end-result on one's own, the resilient person seeks the wisdom and support of others in achieving this.

One of the strategies used in resilience-enhancing interventions is religious coping. This, of course, can only be used for those who have faith in religion or a spiritual outlook. Constructing a personal narrative that gives meaning can assist in developing a healthy perspective on a stressful event, with an impact on overall psychological and physical wellbeing (45).

While psychiatry is most often concerned with protecting the vulnerable person, the flip side of the coin—that is, promoting resilience as a therapeutic and preventive attribute—is increasingly recognized as an important and alternative perspective, particularly when stressor-related disorders are emerging or present (see Box 4.1). It requires a hands-on approach particularly with the person's social network, as this is one of the main building blocks. A clear and accessible approach to resilience-building interventions is outlined by Iacoviello & Charney (46). The focus is on what is positive and provides optimism rather than on the negative, and identifying role models are elements of the treatment. Suitable role models could include others

Box 4.1 Vignette 3: Resilience enhancement

Ms A is a 35-year-old woman who was employed in a small garage/car sales office as a secretary. She worked there for 10 years and saw it as a family business because the wife of the owner had become a close friend through the years. During the recession, Ms A lost her job when the business closed and she saw little hope of ever finding employment again. She was especially upset because this placed a further financial burden on herself and her husband. After losing her job, Ms A began to have feelings of self-doubt about herself. She described symptoms of anxiety and depression and she worried excessively. She withdrew from friends and family and she stopped socializing because she disliked being viewed as somebody who was unemployed. She always had a strong work ethic. She began drinking alcohol excessively a few times each week but never more than three glasses of wine each time. Ordinarily she seldom took alcohol.

Ms A was referred to the outpatient clinic with a diagnosis of 'depression' and had been commenced on an antidepressant. This medication was discontinued and a diagnosis of adjustment disorder was made. The clinician focused on enhancing the resilience of this lady. Cognitive-behavioural strategies were used to re-frame her negative cognitions about herself (as an unemployed women) and the future. She eventually accepted that she was one of many who were unemployed at this time and that it was not her fault that she had been made redundant. She was able to identify others who had come through redundancy and found employment again. She was encouraged to find a resilient role model and she chose the wife of her former employer, who herself had found employment when she lost her position in the company after it closed. Ms A began meeting her regularly for coffee and they discussed how she had coped when she was in a similar position. Sharing their approaches to the problem helped Ms A cope better. The support provided by this lady encouraged Ms A to become more active and to re-engage with tennis, which she had played in the past, and to return to her book club from which she had withdrawn. Her anxiety and depression gradually lessened as Ms A re-engaged with family, friends, and hobbies. She did not require any medication and she found alternative employment 6 months later through a contact in the tennis club.

who have experienced and overcome similar stressors. Confronting fears rather than avoiding them, and attending to one's physical wellbeing, are also important in fostering resilience. Therapies derived from these principles include prolonged exposure therapy (47) and cognitive reprocessing therapy (48).

Conclusions

Little thought has been given to the model underpinning AD. A biological one, a crisis model, a cognitive model, and a stress/trauma model have all been used by different investigators (13, 15, 18, 23). The criteria proposed for ICD-11 (5) are underpinned by the stress/trauma model, with symptoms overlapping with some of those occurring following trauma. The risk factors currently identified are broad and overlap with those found in other psychiatric conditions, although DSM states that AD is usually found in those with no prior psychiatric disorder. The protective factors are likewise similar to those offering protection from disorder, and resilience has received significant attention in recent years. Techniques to enhance this have been developed and are increasingly finding a place in therapy.

References

1. **World Health Organization**. Mental disorders: Glossary and guide to their classification in accordance with the Seventh Revision of the International Classification of Diseases. Albany, NY: World Health Organization; 1955.

2. **World Health Organization**. Mental disorders: Glossary and guide to their classification in accordance with the Eighth Revision of the International Classification of Diseases. Albany, NY: World Health Organization; 1965.

3. **World Health Organization**. Mental disorders: Glossary and guide to their classification in accordance with the Ninth Revision of the International Classification of Diseases. Albany, NY: World Health Organization; 1978.

4. **World Health Organization**. The ICD-10 classification of mental and behavioural disorders: Clinical description and diagnostic guidelines (ICD-10). Geneva: World Health Organization; 1992.

5. **Maercker A, Einsle F, Kollner V.** Adjustment disorders as stress response syndromes: a new diagnostic concept and its exploration in a medical sample. Psychopathology. 2007;**40**(3):135–46.

6. **American Psychiatric Association**. Diagnostic and statistical manual of mental disorders. 1st ed. Washington, DC: American Psychiatric Association; 1952.

7. **American Psychiatric Association**. Diagnostic and statistical manual of mental disorders. 2nd ed. Washington, DC: American Psychiatric Association; 1968.

8. **American Psychiatric Association**. Diagnostic and statistical manual of mental disorders. 3rd ed. Washington, DC: American Psychiatric Association; 1980.

9. **American Psychiatric Association**. Diagnostic and statistical manual of mental disorders. 3rd ed, text revision. Washington, DC: American Psychiatric Association; 1987.

10. **American Psychiatric Association**. Diagnostic and statistical manual of mental disorders. 4th ed. Washington, DC: American Psychiatric Association; 1994.

11. **American Psychiatric Association**. Diagnostic and statistical manual of mental disorders. 5th ed. Washington, DC: American Psychiatric Association; 2013.

12. **Strain J, Diefenbacher A**. The adjustments disorders: the conundrums of the diagnoses. Compr Psychiatry. 2008;**49**:121–30.

13. **Horowitz MJ**. Stress response syndromes: PTSD, grief, and adjustment disorders. 3rd ed. Northvale: Jason Aronson; 1997.

14. **Kübler-Ross, E**. On death and dying. New York: Macmillan; 1969.

15. **Creamer M, Burgess P, Pattison P**. Reaction to trauma: a cognitive processing model. J Abnorm Psychol. 1992;**101**(3):452–9.

16. **Maciejewski PK, Zhang B, Block SD, Prigerson HG**. An empirical examination of the stage theory of grief. JAMA. 2007;**297**(7):716–23.

17. **Lindemann E**. Symptomatology and management of acute grief. Am J Psychiatry. 1994;**101**:141–8.

18. **Caplan G**. Principles of preventive psychiatry. New York: Basic Books; 1964.

19. **Caplan G**. Support systems and community mental health: Lectures on concept development. New York: Behavioral Publications; 1974.

20. **Lazarus RS, Folkman S**. Stress, appraisal and coping. New York: Springer; 1984.

21. **Johnson JH, Sarason IG**. Recent developments in research on life stress. In: Hamilton V and Warburton DM, editors. Human stress and cognition: an information processing approach. New York: John Wiley; 1979. p. 205–36.

22. **Felsten G**. Stress reactivity and vulnerability to depressed mood in college students. Pers Individ Dif. 2004;**36**:789–800.

23. **Selye H**. The stress of life. New York, NY: McGraw-Hill; 1956.

24. **Strain J, Friedman MJ**. Considering adjustment disorders as stress response syndromes for DSM-5. Depress Anxiety. 2011;**28**(9):818–23.

25. **Bruffaerts R, Sabbe M, Demyttenaere K**. Attenders of a university hospital psychiatric emergency services in Belgium—general characteristics and gender differences. Soc Psychiatry Psychiatr Epidemiol. 2004;**39**(2):146–53.

26. **Despland JN, Monod L, Ferrero F.** Clinical relevance of adjustment disorder in DSM-III-R and DSM-IV. Compr Psychiatry. 1995;**36**(6):454–60.

27. **Doherty AM, Jabbar F, Kelly BD, Casey P.** Distinguishing between adjustment disorder and depressive episode in clinical practice: the role of personality disorder. J Affect Disord. 2014;**168**:78–85.

28. **For-Wey L, Lee F-Y, Shu B-C.** The premorbid personality in military students with adjustment disorder. Mil Psychol. 2006;**18**(1):77–88.

29. **Na K-S, Oh S-J, Jung H-Y, Lee SI, Kim Y-K, Han C, et al.** Temperament and character of young male conscripts with adjustment disorder: a case-control study. J Nerv Ment Dis. 2012;**200**(11):973–7.

30. **Connor-Smith JK, Flachsbart C.** Relations between personality and coping: a meta-analysis. J Pers Soc Psychol. 2007;**93**(6):1080–107.

31. **For-Wey L, Fei-Yin L, Bih-Ching S.** The relationship between life adjustment and parental bonding in military personnel with adjustment disorder in Taiwan. Mil Med. 2002;**167**(8):678–82.

32. **Vallejo-Sánchez B, Pérez-García AM.** The role of personality and coping in adjustment disorder. Clin Psychol. 2015. doi:10.1111/cp.12064

33. **Horn AB, Maercker A.** (Anpassung an ein belastendes Ereignis im Paar: Depressionen beim Partner als Risiko für das Auftreten von Anpassungsstörungen). Adjustment to a stressful event in the couple: depression of the partner as risk for adjustment disorder. Psychother Psychosom Med Psychol. 2015;**65**(8):296–303.

34. **Furukawa TA, Harai H, Hirai T, Kitamura T, Takahashi K.** Social Support Questionnaire among psychiatric patients with various diagnoses and normal controls. Soc Psychiatry Psychiatr Epidemiol. 1999;**34**(4):216–22.

35. **Chen P-F, Chen C-S, Chen C-C, Lung F-W.** Alexithymia as a screening index for male conscripts with adjustment disorder. Psychiatr Q. 2011;**82**(2):139–50.

36. **Fankhauser S, Wagner B, Krammer S, Aeschbach M, Pepe A, Maercker A, et al.** The impact of social and interpersonal resources on adjustment disorder symptoms in older age: motivational variables as mediators? GeroPsych. 2010;**23**(4):227–41.

37. **Giotakos O.** Parenting received in childhood and early separation anxiety in male conscripts with adjustment disorder. Mil Med. 2002;**167**(1):28–33.

38. **Polyakova I, Knobler HY, Ambrumova A, Lerner V.** Characteristics of suicidal attempts in major depression versus adjustment reactions. J Affect Disord. 1998;**47**:159–67.

39. **Paykel ES, Klerman GL, Prusoff BA.** Personality and symptom pattern in depression. Br J Psychiatry. 1976;**129**:327–34.

40 **Benjaminsen S.** Primary non-endogenous depression and features attributed to reactive depression. J Affect Disord. 1981;**3**(2):245–59.

41. **Coryell W, Winokur G, Maser JD.** Recurrently situational (reactive) depression: a study of course, phenomenology and familial psychopathology. J Affect Disord.1994;**31**(3):203–10.

42. **Southwick SM, Charney DS.** The science of resilience: implications for the prevention and treatment of depression. Science. 2012;**338**(6103):79–82.

43. **Connor KM, Davidson JRT.** Development of a new resilience scale: the Connor-Davidson Resilience Scale (CD-RISC). Depress Anxiety. 2003;**18**:76–82.

44. **Carver CS, Scheier MF, Segerstrom SC.** Optimism. Clin Psychol Rev. 2010;**30**:879–89.

45. **Pargament KI, Koenig HG, Tarakeshwar N, Hahn J.** Religious coping methods as predictors of psychological, physical and spiritual outcomes among medically ill elderly patients: a two-year longitudinal study. J Health Psychol. 2004;**9**:713–30.

46. **Iacoviello BM, Charney DS.** Therapeutic adaptations of resilience: helping patients overcome the effects of trauma and stress. In: Trauma and stressor-related disorders: A handbook for clinicians. Casey P and Strain JJ, editors. Arlington, VA: American Psychiatric Publications, American Psychiatric Association; 2016.

47. **Williams M, Cahill S, Foa E.** Psychotherapy for post-traumatic stress disorder. In: Stein D, Hollander E and Rothbaum B, editors. Textbook of anxiety disorders. 2nd ed. Arlington, VA: American Psychiatric Publishing; 2010. p. 603–27.

48. **Resick PA, Schnicke MK.** Cognitive processing therapy for rape victims: A treatment manual. Newbury Park, CA: Sage; 1993.

Chapter 5

The biological basis
of adjustment disorders

Anne Doherty

Introduction

There is a striking paucity of published research concerning the biological basis of adjustment disorder (AD). There are very few studies
examining the genetic, neuroimaging, or neurochemical predictors of
this commonly diagnosed (in clinical practice) condition. While there
is a scarcity of biological studies on (AD), the few that exist demonstrate distinctions between AD and major depression. This is most
marked in those studies which examine the hypothalamo-pituitary-
adrenal (HPA) axis in those with AD and major depression who ex-
press suicidal ideation or present with suicidal behaviours.

Despite the prevalent belief that AD is a mild 'sub-syndrome', it
is associated with high rates of suicidal behaviour: 25–60% (1, 2).
It has been implicated in up to one-third of completed suicides on
psychological autopsy (3), and it is suggested that it is the condition
most commonly associated with suicidal behaviour in the developing
world (4). Polyakova et al. suggested that there may be differences
between AD and major depression in psychological risk variables
and sociodemographic profile (5). The biological data suggests that
there may be some differences in the biological risk variables for the
two conditions. These differences are likely to become more prominent as the conceptualization of AD evolves in ICD-11 (International
Classification of Diseases, Eleventh Revision), where there is a shift
in the conceptualization of AD to a condition more akin to post-
traumatic stress disorder (PTSD), another condition which requires
the presence of stressor (6).

The few studies that report biological data on AD have small datasets, and most are conducted in consultation-liaison psychiatry settings. Given the strong association between AD and both suicidal behaviours and completed suicide, it seems surprising that there are so few biological studies on a disorder which is most commonly found in the most biological of psychiatry settings (consultation-liaison psychiatry in acute medical hospitals).

Genetics

There has been little scientific exploration of any relationship between adjustment disorders and genetic factors. There is evidence that individuals with polymorphism of the serotonin transporter gene are more vulnerable to developing mood disorders when under stress, and have an increased cortisol response to awakening, which may be inhibited in healthy people by prefrontal serotonergic neurotransmission [7].

Geijer et al. conducted a study of a Swedish cohort of patients who presented with suicidal behaviours, comprising 165 patients, 37 of whom had a diagnosis of AD, and 99 healthy controls. They examined polymorphisms in the genes coding for tryptophan hydroxylase (TPH), serotonin 2a ($5HT_{2A}$), and serotonin transporter (SERT) [8]. It was found that there were non-significant differences in the expression of the TPH a-allele in those who presented with suicidal behaviours compared to controls, and that this was most markedly seen in AD (but remained non-significant). No significant differences were observed in the expression of $5HT_{2A}$ and SERT among those who presented with suicidal behaviours and controls, or between the diagnostic groups.

Strain & Friedman have suggested that further study of gene/environment interactions in adjustment disorders is required to examine the role of biology and environment in vulnerability and resilience in AD compared with similar psychiatric conditions [9].

Neuroimaging

AD, unlike many other psychiatric disorders, has attracted very little neuroimaging research. One study which examined MRI (magnetic resonance imaging) scans in a cohort of 25 Taiwanese conscripts who had been diagnosed with AD by means of a 'M.I.N.I.' semi-structured interview (the Mini International Neuropsychiatric Interview), and compared them to 25 matched healthy controls, found decreased grey matter in the right medial frontal gyrus of the medial prefrontal cortex in the participants with AD (10). The medial prefrontal cortex has a role in the extinction of learned fear, and it is possible that with decreased tissue in this area the process of down-regulating fear is impaired, resulting in maladaptive behaviours in fear-inducing scenarios, and may predispose an individual to developing AD.

The authors speculate that given that the medial prefrontal cortex may be associated with stress-induced anxiety and depressive symptoms, abnormalities in this region may predict the development of such symptoms in response to stress (11). Reduced medial pre-frontal cortex volume is associated with deficits in executive function (12). Executive function refers to flexible, goal-directed cognitive function and includes abilities such as working memory, problem solving, planning, and attentional control. As executive dysfunction is associated with demonstrable difficulty in adapting to unfamiliar or stressful situations, it may be regarded as a barrier to healthy or adaptive coping (13).

The sole study of AD that utilized 18F-fluorodeoxyglucosepositron emission topography (PET) scans, and which examined patients with a recent diagnosis of cancer and either AD or depression, found that prior to the development of psychiatric symptoms, patients had evidence of decreased metabolism in the right medial frontal gyrus and increased metabolism in the right posterior cingulate, right anterior cingulate, left subcallosal, and left caudate cortices (14). This study, however, did not examine the risk factors for either major depression or AD, and its findings do not allow a distinction to be made between those disorders on this basis. Therefore, we cannot use this finding to make a prognostic judgement regarding those episodes (AD) that may be self-limiting, requiring supportive treatment only, and those that are not self-limiting (major depression) and require specific treatment.

Godinez at al. conducted a functional MRI study of twins where one of each twin pair only had been exposed to significant life events, although they did not examine psychiatric diagnoses or symptoms (15).

They found that twins that had experienced multiple, severe stressful life events showed greater activation of the limbic system regions throughout the task than their control co-twins.

The HPA axis

Selye was one of the first to comment on the role of the HPA axis in stress responses, in 1956 (16). Since that time, although much research has been conducted into the role of the HPA axis in depression and anxiety, little has been conducted with specific reference to AD. Lindqvist et al. examined serum cortisol levels and suicidality among individuals who presented following attempted suicide (17). They found differences between AD and major depression on the dexamethasone suppression test in individuals who were admitted to hospital following presentation with attempted suicide. This study of 39 individuals with AD and 39 with a diagnosis of major depression (according to clinical diagnosis by two psychiatrists) found that individuals with AD showed a positive correlation between suicidal intent (as measured by the suicide intent scale, where a higher score indicates a greater degree of suicidality) and post-dexamethasone cortisol, although this difference was not significant. Those individuals with major depression, however, showed a significant negative correlation between post-dexamethasone serum cortisol and suicidal intent. The authors suggested that the more rapid progression of symptoms in AD compared with major depression may explain some of the differences between the two groups (17).

This study by Lindqvist et al. confirmed the findings of an earlier study by Tripodianakis et al. of neurochemical variables in 53 patients with suicidal behaviour and AD who were admitted to a Greek hospital. Clinical diagnosis was used and this study found significant elevation of cortisol levels compared to (n = 50) healthy controls (18).

Banki et al. studied 141 female patients, 24 of whom had a clinical diagnosis of AD, and found a comparable degree of dexamethasone non-suppression in both AD (71%) and major depression (82%). Of note, in this study the greatest proportion of individuals who had presented with suicidal attempts had a diagnosis of AD, and across diagnostic categories those who presented with violent and non-violent suicidal acts had higher levels of non-suppression than those who presented without suicide attempts (19).

Another study conducted by Rocco et al. examined cortisol levels in 48 individuals with a clinical diagnosis of AD precipitated by workplace stress. This study reported an inverse relationship between morning cortisol levels and psychasthenia & depression scores on the Minnesota Multiphasic Personality Inventory (MMPI) (20). Unlike previous studies which examined cortisol suppression in major depression, this study found that in AD the dexamethasone suppression test was normal, thus resulting in a similar profile to other stress-related conditions such as PTSD and chronic fatigue syndrome. The authors suggest that with further research, a cortisol 'cut-off' might perhaps be agreed for the diagnosis of AD (20). If this were validated it could be a useful test for distinguishing between AD and major depression.

The few studies which examined the HPA axis in AD have mostly examined individuals who presented with suicidal behaviours. Although there are few studies exploring this area, they consistently suggest that while individuals with major depression have an unusual stress response, those with AD have a similar pattern to the normal stress response seen in healthy individuals, which supports the dominant understanding of AD being a stress-related condition. This suggests that there are key differences in the pathophysiological processes between major depression and AD, and that it may be possible to distinguish between AD based on cortisol responses.

Neurotransmitters and monoamine theory

Monoamine oxidase (MAO) is the primary enzyme of monoamine oxidation, and is found in the outer membrane of mitochondria in various cells. The two subtypes, MAO-A and MAO-B, are responsible for the catabolism of dopamine, tyramine, and tryptamine, while serotonin, noradrenaline, and adrenaline are catabolized by MAO-A, and phenethylamine and benzylamine by MAO-B. Owing to their direct role in the de-activation of neurotransmitters, they have been associated with a range of psychiatric and neurological disorders. While considerable research has been conducted into the role of monoamines in major depression, there have been merely a handful of studies which have examined the role of monoamines in AD.

Banki et al. examined 141 female patients, of whom 24 had a clinical diagnosis of AD (the remainder had diagnoses of major depression, psychosis, or alcohol dependence). Cerebrospinal fluid (CSF) samples were obtained by lumbar puncture and levels of 5-hydroxyindoleacetic acid (5-HIAA, a metabolite of serotonin) and homovanillic acid (HVA, a metabolite of dopamine) were measured. Those who presented with violent suicide attempts demonstrated lower levels of 5-HIAA across the four diagnostic groups, with no significant differences across the diagnoses. CSF levels of HVA were found to be lower in those individuals who had presented with violent suicide attempts: again, there were no significant differences between the diagnoses (19).

Tripodianakis et al. examined MAO activity in 53 hospital inpatients with suicidal behaviour and a clinical diagnosis of AD (18). In addition to finding elevated cortisol levels in AD compared to controls (n = 50), platelet MAO activity was found to be significantly lower in patients with AD than in controls. This study revealed that there were significantly higher levels of urinary 3-methoxy-4-hydroxyphenylglycol (MHPG, a noradrenaline metabolite) in patients with AD than in controls. However, there were no significant differences in levels of urinary 5-HIAA, a serotonin metabolite, or HVA, a catecholamine metabolite, between patients and controls. In addition, significant differences in platelet MAO activity were found in patients with AD versus controls, with the individuals with a diagnosis of AD demonstrating lower levels of activity than the controls (18). Previous studies which examined MHPG in people with depression who presented with suicidal behaviour had found that these groups have overall lower MHPG excretion rates than healthy controls (21), although high levels of urinary MHPG have been reported in previous studies of anxiety disorders (22).

An earlier study by Tripodianakis et al. had examined platelet MAO activity in 82 patients who had been hospitalized following attempted suicide and had had a diagnosis of AD, dysthymia, or personality disorder (23). This study found significantly lower levels of platelet MAO activity in individuals who had presented following a suicide attempt. No significant difference was found in platelet MAO activity between patients with AD (n = 33) and controls, but the platelet MAO activity in the patients with AD was more similar to that seen in healthy controls than that seen in dysthymia or personality disorder: both groups showed marked lowering of MAO activity (23).

Given the limited evidence that monoamine activity may be associated with AD, there may be a potential role for medications that directly influence neurotransmitter activity in the management of AD. However, the evidence for the use of antidepressant agents that directly influence neurotransmitters is weak. Overall, the evidence for antidepressants in AD remains unclear. There is, at present, an ongoing Cochrane Systematic Review focusing on double-blind, randomized controlled trials which is examining the quality of the evidence in terms of the benefit of antidepressants, anxiolytics, and other agents (24).

Much of the evidence in the management of adjustment disorders is focused on psychological therapies or on pharmacological symptomatic management rather than pharmacotherapies that have a direct effect on neurotransmitters. Antidepressants are often used in clinical practice, despite the limited evidence base (25).

One retrospective study in a primary care setting found that individuals with AD may be twice as likely to improve on selective serotonin reuptake inhibitors (SSRIs) as individuals with major depression on SSRIs. As this is a retrospective chart-based study, it is difficult to ascertain whether this reflects the natural course of AD with its high rate of spontaneous remission, or perhaps direct pharmacological effects of the medications used (26).

Ansseau et al., in a double-blind, multicentre study which compared mianserin (a tetracyclic antidepressant), tianeptine (a psychotropic with antidepressant and anxiolytic properties), and alprazolam (a short-acting benzodiazepine) in 152 patients with AD with mixed symptoms (anxiety and depression) found very similar efficacy of antidepressant and anxiolytic properties of the three medications used (27). Similarly, Razavi et al. suggest that in individuals with cancer who develop AD with symptoms of anxiety and depression, trazadone (an antidepressant with serotonin antagonism and reuptake inhibition properties) may be *more* beneficial than benzodiazepines (28).

Given the paucity and heterogeneity of these studies it is difficult to use them to draw any conclusions about any direct effect of SSRIs or other medication on any underlying neurobiological mechanism in AD.

Pain theory and other biological theories of adjustment disorder

Bar et al. conducted a study examining pain responses in AD (29). They reported that participants with an acute presentation of AD with depressed mood (precipitated by an interpersonal crisis) demonstrated an overall increased threshold for pain compared with a control group. Specifically, they found that all parameters (thermal, electrical) investigated were significantly increased on the right-hand side of the body, whereas, pain parameters did not differ from controls on the left-hand side, although a trend towards increased threshold was noted. Scores on the Hamilton depression rating scale (HAM-D) that measured depressive symptoms were positively correlated to thermal pain threshold parameters on the right arm, and there was a marked reduction in pain sensitivity. Thus, there was a correlation between the severity of the depressive symptoms in AD and the degree of pain threshold disturbance.

Although the authors were unable to identify the mechanism for the decreased sensitivity to pain in AD, they observed a similarity to the previously reported response to pain in major depression: four previous studies had reported hypoalgesia in major depression. Unlike patients with major depression, however, those studied with AD had been symptomatic for a brief period only. The authors concluded that a better understanding of the pain response might be useful in our future understanding of the physiology of AD (29).

Brundin et al. reported statistically significant lower levels of orexin (a neurotransmitter regulating arousal, wakefulness, and appetite which is produced in the hypothalamus) in the CSF of individuals with a diagnosis of major depression (n = 31) who presented with suicidal behaviours than in the CSF of those with a diagnosis of AD (n = 23) (30). Orexin levels correlated significantly with CSF levels of somatostatin and corticotropin-releasing factor. The authors suggest that this may indicate a hypothalamic neurobiological distinction between the two diagnostic groups. The authors also examined specific symptoms associated with reduced orexin and found that higher scores on measures of lassitude, slowness of movement, and global rating of illness were significantly associated with lower CSF orexin levels (31).

The authors did not report whether there were any distinguishing factors between the diagnostic groups with respect to these symptoms.

A pilot study conducted by Di Rosa et al. examined levels of nitrated and carbonylated proteins in people who developed an adjustment disorder in the context of work-related bullying (32). The presence of nitrated and carbonylated proteins is a marker of oxidative stress conditions, and elevated levels of these proteins are seen across a range of severe pathological conditions from Alzheimer's disease to acute respiratory distress syndrome. Oxidative stress conditions are associated with consequences including tissue damage and disease progression, and the presence of nitrated and carbonylated proteins may be considered a proxy for oxidation and may therefore have a function in the monitoring of disease progression (33).

Di Rosa et al.'s study recruited 19 people with AD and compared them to 38 healthy controls. They found that other stress markers, including levels of protein carbonyl groups and of nitrosylated proteins, are significantly higher in those victims of workplace bullying than in healthy individuals (33). This suggests that AD precipitates an oxidative stress reaction in affected individuals. The authors hypothesized that exogenous antioxidants, and indeed adrenaline and noradrenaline, may protect macromolecules from such oxidative processes, and that the progression of depression may potentiate the oxidation triggered by stress related to life events.

Andreasen & Wasek found an association between a diagnosis of AD and paternal substance abuse disorder, and reported rates of 11.8% for adults and as high as 21.6% in adolescents studied (34). However, there is no evidence that personal alcohol abuse is a predictor of AD (35). Therefore, it seems likely that alcohol use is related to AD by mediation of psychological factors in early life, and there is no convincing evidence of a direct biological relationship between either personal or paternal alcohol use and AD.

Why are there so few studies into the biological basis of adjustment disorder?

The lack of adequate biological research into this common diagnosis is striking given the frequency with which AD is diagnosed in clinical practice, and given the fact that in certain settings such as emergency departments and acute hospitals it is more common than major depression (36). As AD has been identified as a significant risk factor for suicidal behaviours and completed suicide (1–3), surely it warrants further scientific exploration?

Certainly, very few studies have been published in the area. Does this reflect a publication bias arising from the controversies attached to this diagnosis? Is this a consequence of the difficulty in obtaining funding for research studies in AD? Perhaps it is because several biologically focused researchers have dismissed this diagnostic category based on the instability of the diagnosis and the controversy that has accompanied this diagnostic category through its evolution throughout the twentieth century (37, 38).

Although AD has a strong association with suicidal ideation and behaviours, much of the research into suicidality grew out of the research into suicidality in major depression, and has focused on categories which are adequately covered by the existing semi-structured diagnostic instruments and can thus be more easily researched. Perhaps the neglect of this area of research reflects the difficulties in establishing a standardized diagnosis given the deficiencies of semi-structured interview schedules such as SCID (the Structured Clinical Interview for DSM-IV) and SCAN (the Schedule for Clinical Assessment in Neuropsychiatry), which do not accurately diagnose AD.

In general terms, structured interviews are not helpful in diagnosing AD, as they either do not include it at all, or, as in SCAN, they include it in an appendix under 'Inferences and Attributions', only to be considered if the patient does not meet the criteria for another mental disorder. These schedules are limited in that they diagnose by symptom count, disregarding context. As many patients with AD may have significant symptoms, many of these schedules will diagnose either major depression or an anxiety disorder. This disregard for context and diagnosis of depression once a symptom threshold is reached may explain the absence of AD from the findings of the major epidemiological studies. Many studies focusing on the biological aspects of AD have chosen clinical diagnosis as the gold standard above structured instrument (18–20, 23). With the imminent publication of ICD-11 (International Classification of Diseases, Eleventh Revision), there is a shift in the conceptualization of AD to a condition more akin to PTSD: it remains to be seen whether this will alter how biological research into this condition is conducted.

Strain & Friedman have suggested that future areas for research might include comparison of HPA-axis function both among AD subtypes and with their related diagnostic category (e.g. AD with anxiety symptoms with generalized anxiety disorder) (9). There are further gaps in our knowledge regarding the biological basis of AD: the other areas of neuroimaging, genetics, monoamines, and pain theory all warrant further study.

References

1. Kryzhananovskaya L, Canterbury R. Suicidal behaviour in patients with adjustment disorders. Crisis. 2001;22:125–31.

2. Pelkonen M, Marttunen MJ, Henriksson MM, Lonnqvist JK. Suidality in adjustment disorder—clinical characteristics of adolescent outpatients. Eur Child Adolesc Psychiatry. 2005;14:174–80.

3. Lonnqvist JK, Henriksson MM, Isometsa ET, Marttunen MJ, Heikkinen ME, Aro HM, et al. Mental disorders and suicide prevention. Psychiatry Clin Neurosci 1995;49(suppl 1): S111–16.

4. Manoranjitham SD, Rajkumar AP, Thangadurai P, Prasad J, Jayakaran R, Jacob KS. Risk factors for suicide in rural south India. Br J Psychiatry. 2009;196:26–30.

5. Polyakova I, Knobler HY, Ambrumova A. Characteristics of suicidal attempts in major depression versus adjustment reactions. J Affect Disord. 1998;47:159–67.

6. Bachem R, Perkonigg A, Stein DJ, Maercker A. Measuring the ICD-11 adjustment disorder concept: validity and sensitivity to change of the Adjustment Disorder—New Module questionnaire in a clinical intervention study. Int J Methods Psychiatr Res. 2016;9. [Epub ahead of print]

7. Frokjaer VG, Erritzoe D, Jensen PS, Madsen J, Baaré W, Knudsen GM. Prefrontal serotonin transporter availability is positively associated with the cortisol awakening response. Eur Neuropsychopharmacol. 2012;23:285–94.

8. Geijer T, Frisch A, Persson ML, Wasserman D, Rockah R, Michaelovsky E, et al. Search for association between suicide attempt and serotonergic polymorphisms. Psychiatr Genet. 2000;10:19–26.

9. Strain JJ, Friedman MJ. Considering adjustment disorders as stress response syndromes for DSM-5. Depress Anxiety 2011;28:818–23.

10. Myung W, Na KS, Ham BJ, Oh SJ, Ahn HW, Jung HY. Decreased medial frontal gyrus in patients with adjustment disorder. J Affect Disord. 2016;191:36–40.

11. Long J, Huang X, Liao Y, Hu X, Hu J, Lui S, et al. Prediction of post-earthquake depressive and anxiety symptoms: a longitudinal resting-state fMRI study. Sci Rep. 2014;**4**:6423.

12. Arnsten AFT. Stress signalling pathways that impair prefrontal cortex structure and function. Nat Rev Neurosci. 2009;**10**:410–22.

13. Rodríguez Villegas AL, Salvador Cruz J. Executive functioning and adaptive coping in healthy adults. Appl Neuropsychol Adult. 2015;**22**:124–31.

14. Kumano H, Ida I, Oshima A, Takahashi K, Yuuki N, Amanuma M, et al. Brain metabolic changes associated with predisposition to onset of major depressive disorder and adjustment disorder in cancer patients—a preliminary PET study. J Psychiatr Res. 2007;**41**:591–9.

15. Godinez DA, McRae K, Andrews-Hanna JR, Smolker H, Banich MT. Differences in frontal and limbic brain activation in a small sample of monozygotic twin pairs discordant for severe stressful life events. Neurobiol Stress. 2016;**5**:26–36.

16. Selye, H. The stress of life. New York: McGraw-Hill; 1956.

17. Lindqvist D, Traskman-Bendz L, Vang F. Suicidal intent and the HPA-axis characteristics of suicide attempters with major depressive disorder and adjustment disorders. Arch Suicide Res 2008;**12**:197–207.

18. Tripodianakis J, Markianos M, Sarantidis D, Leotsakou L. Neurochemical variables in subjects with adjustment disorder after suicide attempts. Eur Psychiatry. 2000;**15**:190–5.

19. Banki CS, Arato M, Papp Z, Kurcz M. Biochemical markers in suicidal patients. Investigations with cerebrospinal fluid amine metabolites and neuroendocrine tests. J Affect Disord. 1984;**6**:341–50.

20. Rocco, A, Martocchia A, Frugoni P, Baldini R, Sani G, Di Simone Di Giuseppe B, et al. Inverse correlation between morning plasma cortisol levels and MMPI psychasthenia and depression scale scores in victims of mobbing with adjustment disorders. Neuro Endocrinol Lett. 2007;**28**:610–13.

21. Secunda S, Cross C, Koslow S, Katz MM, Kocsis J, Maas JW, et al. Biochemistry and suicidal behavior in depressed patients. Biol Psychiatry. 1986;**21**:756–67.

22. Beckmann H, Goodwin FK. Urinary MHPG in subgroups of depressed patients and normal controls. Neuropsychobiology. 1980;**6**:90–1.

23. Tripodianakis J, Markianos M, Sarantidis D, Istikoglou C, Andara A, Bistolaki E. Platelet monoamine oxidase in attempted suicide. Relations to sex, psychiatric diagnosis, mode of attempt, and previous attempts. Eur Psychiatry. 1995;**10**:44–8.

24. Casey P, Pillay D, Wilson L, Maercker A, Rice A, Kelly BK. Pharmacological interventions for adjustment disorders in adults (Protocol). Cochrane Database Syst Rev. 2013; Issue 6. Art No.: CD010530. DOI: 10.1002/14651858

25. Stewart JW, Quitkin FM, Klein DF. The pharmacotherapy of minor depression. Am J Psychother. 1992;**46**:23–36.

26. Hameed U, Schwartz TL, Malhotra K, West RL, Bertone F. Antidepressant treatment in the primary care office: outcomes for adjustment disorder versus major depression. Ann Clin Psychiatry. 2005;**17**:77–81.

27. Ansseau M, Bataille M, Briole G, de Nayer A, Fauchère PA, Ferrero F, et al. Controlled comparison of tianeptine, alprazolam and mianserin in the treatment of ADs with depression and anxiety. Hum Psychopharmacol. 1996;**11**:293–8.

28. Razavi D, Kormoss N, Collard A, Farvacques C, Delvaux N. Comparative study of the efficacy and safety of trazodone versus clorazepate in the treatment of adjustment disorders in cancer patients: a pilot study. J Int Med Res. 1999;**27**:264–72.

29. Bar KJ, Brehm S, Boettger MK, Wagner G, Boettger S, Sauer H. Decreased sensitivity to experimental pain in adjustment disorder. Eur J Pain. 2006;**10**:467–71.

30. Brundin L, Bjorkqvist M, Petersen A, Traskman-Bendz L. Reduced orexin levels in the cerebrospinal fluid of suicidal patients with major depressive disorder. Eur Neuropsychopharmacol. 2007;**17**:573–9.

31. Brundin L, Bjorkqvist M, Petersen A, Traskman-Bendz L. Orexin and psychiatric symptoms in suicide attempters. J Affect Disord. 2007;**100**:259–63.

32. Di Rosa AE, Gangemi S, Cristani M, Fenga C, Saitta S, Abenavoli E, et al. Serum levels of carbonylated and nitrosylated proteins in mobbing victims with workplace adjustment disorders. Biol Psychol. 2009;**82**:308–11.

33. Dalle-Donne I, Giustarini DI, Colombo R, Rossi R, Milzani A. Protein carbonylation in human diseases. Trends Mol Med. 2003;**9**:169–76.

34. Andreasen NC, Wasek P. Adjustment disorders in adolescents and adults. Arch Gen Psychiatry. 1980;**37**:1166–70.

35. Breslow RE, Klinger BI, Erickson BJ. Acute intoxication and substance abuse among patients presenting to a psychiatric emergency service. Gen Hosp Psychiatry. 1996;**18**:183–91.

36. Silverstone PH. Prevalence of psychiatric disorders in medical inpatients. J Nerv Ment Dis. 1996;**184**:43–51.

37. Arbabi M Laghaveepoor R, Golestan B, Mahdanian A, Nejatisafa A, Tavakkoli A, et al. Diagnoses, requests and timings of 503 consultations in two general hospitals. Acta Med Iran. 2012;**50**:53–60.

38. Carta MG, Balestrien M, Murru A, Hardoy MC. Adjustment disorder: epidemiology, diagnosis and treatment. Clin Pract Epidemiol Ment Health. 2009;**26**:5–15.

Chapter 6

Making the diagnosis in clinical practice

Patricia Casey

Adjustment disorder (AD) is classified in section F43 (Reactions to severe stress, and adjustment disorders) in ICD-10 (International Classification of Diseases, Tenth Revision) (1). Post-traumatic stress disorder (PTSD) and acute stress disorder are also included in this section.

The diagnosis of AD is a clinical one, as in almost all psychiatric disorders. But this is more difficult for AD than for other psychiatric disorders, for a number of reasons. These include:

- the absence of diagnostic criteria in DSM-5 (2) and ICD-10 (3) other than the requirement for a stressor
- the subthreshold status of AD in ICD-10 and DSM-5, precluding it as a diagnosis when the criteria for another disorder are met (see Box 6.3)
- the absence of guidance on what constitutes a normal, as distinct from a pathological, reaction to a stressor
- the neglect of AD in research as a consequence of the above
- the longitudinal nature of the diagnosis, which requires prediction at time 1 that symptoms will resolve spontaneously when the stressor or its consequences are modified/removed by time 2.

McHugh & Slavney (3) point to the challenges facing those making psychiatric diagnoses, in general. While the ICD and DSM diagnostic manuals emphasize this when applying diagnostic criteria and point to the importance of a detailed clinical history and information gathering from multiple sources, these authors are concerned that the diagnostic exercise is now cursory and based on the Procrustean tick-box approach (3). This concern has a particular resonance when applied to the diagnostic process in respect of AD, where clinical skills and nuance are essential in distinguishing AD from other overlapping conditions. There is evidence to support the dangers alluded to above from studies that compare the clinical with the research diagnosis of AD. Research diagnoses are, by their nature, made in a sterile manner, applying the diagnostic criteria without context so as to avoid the vagaries of personal judgement. There is poor concordance for the diagnosis of AD and major depression, with AD diagnosed clinically more often than major depression, yet when diagnostic instruments such as SCAN (Schedule for Clinical Assessment in Neuropsychiatry) are used, the proportions are reversed (4, 5).

A step-by-step guide to making a clinical diagnosis of AD will be presented in this chapter. It should be read in conjunction with Chapter 3.

Risk factors

The risk factors for AD are no different from those for other psychiatric disorders. In particular, the association between aspects of personality and AD, which is intuitively appealing, has not been supported by research since personality disorder, per se, is higher in those meeting criteria for depressive episode than AD (6). That is not to say that more dimensional aspects of personality, such as neuroticism (5) and self-directedness (7), are not important, but that in themselves they are not specific to AD. While ICD-10 (1) comments on the role of personal vulnerability, ICD-11 (8) is silent on this. In any event it is not clear whether this even refers to personality or some other inter-personal risk factor such as poor support or isolation. DSM-5 (2) does not refer to vulnerability either. Thus, while personality should be assessed, as it should be in any psychiatric evaluation, it should not of itself determine the diagnostic label. These matters are discussed further in Chapter 4, pp. 57–9).

Stressful events are common, and exposure to these is part of everyday life. Their salience for the individual depends on the perspective of that person, and there is huge personal variation in this.

For some, a minor stressor such as the break-up of a recently formed relationship might result in significant distress and/or self-harm, while for others a major event such as a divorce, while upsetting, might also provide relief. Context is also important: losing a job for one person might lead to debt and emotionally devastating consequences, while for another it might be perceived as freedom to do other things such as returning to education or pursuing a new career. Thus the personal relevance of the stressor is important when considering AD. Along with this, the support systems that are available to a person at time of distress and crisis are relevant also and, as in other disorders, positive support strengthens the individual's resilience.

Cultural factors will also play a role; this is particularly so in response to grief. For example, the displays of breast beating and wailing that are normal in some cultures would be considered excessive by western European standards, and a diagnosis of AD would be inappropriate in circumstances in which breast-beating is normal. So, various personal, historical, psychosocial, and cultural factors are likely to modify or accentuate the response to a stressor and will determine whether the reaction to the event is normal and adaptive or pathological.

The stressor: psychosocial or traumatic?

A stressor is an essential requirement: the diagnosis of AD cannot be made in the absence of this. Other conditions can also be triggered following exposure to a stressor, and there is evidence that over 80% of those diagnosed with major depression/depressive episode (DE) have experienced a recent life event, but unlike AD, this is not essential (9). It is accepted that once DE has occurred the person will thereafter be vulnerable to non-triggered episodes, while in the context of AD there is little evidence regarding the sensitizing role of previous AD to other disorders in the future, yet O'Donnell et al. (10) found that of those diagnosed with AD following serious injuries, 20% developed other disorders subsequently. However, owing to methodological issues, other explanations might also be offered for this and the finding needs replication.

The type of stressor is not specifically stated by either set of criteria, unlike that required to make a diagnosis of PTSD, where it has to be one that is traumatic—that is, an event that is perceived and experienced as a threat to one's safety or to the stability of one's world.

For AD, DSM-5 states that the stressor can be of any type, although there is some evidence that events relating to marital difficulties are the most common in those with AD compared to those with major depression (9), and while statistically significant, this is not likely to be clinically helpful since a gamut of stressors can cause AD, including those that are traumatic. DSM-IV (11) specifically required a psycho-social stressor; this was changed simply to a 'stressor' in DSM-IV-TR (DSM-IV, text revision) (12) since it was recognized that not all stressors were psychosocial (e.g., serious physical illness), and this broad term has been retained in DSM-5 (2).

There is now evidence that even stressors normally associated with PTSD, such as living in a war-torn country, being a refugee, or being involved in a serious traffic accident can lead to AD rather than PTSD (13). Similarly, after a traumatic event, such as being the victim of an assault, the full criteria for PTSD may not be met. In DSM-IV this was labelled as AD; in DSM-5 it will be placed in the 'Other Specified Trauma and Stressor-related Disorders' category.

ICD-10 (1) excludes unusual or catastrophic events as possible triggers for AD, and symptoms following such events that do not meet the full criteria for PTSD are not discussed in the document. Strict adherence to the criteria should preclude them from being diagnosed as AD, although in clinical practice they usually are.

In ICD-11, it is unclear whether subthreshold PTSD will be included in the AD diagnostic group or in a subtype of PTSD, as in DSM-5. A further area of uncertainty regarding the application of the proposed ICD-11 criteria is the requirement that the trigger must be psychosocial or an event leading to life changes. Not all stressors are psychosocial or life-changing, and by specifying these, some abnormal reactions occurring in response to, for example, a minor road traffic accident, might be excluded. It remains to be seen how this will be resolved.

Onset and duration

The shorter the latency between the occurrence of the stressor and the onset of symptoms, the greater the likelihood that the event has a causal role. The time specifier of 1 month in ICD-10, and 3 months in DSM-5, is not based on any firm evidence. It is this author's opinion that the 3-month time gap in DSM-5 is, ordinarily, excessive unless there are consequences to the stressor that take several months to develop—for example, aspects of physical injury post-accident that deflect from the psychological impact. The more temporally remote the stressor is from the onset of symptoms, the greater the risk of false attribution of symptoms to the event. Under these circumstances the symptoms might be better explained by major depression/depressive episode than by AD, and treated accordingly. DSM-5 does allow for the onset of symptoms more than 3 months after a stressor and has termed these 'adjustment-like disorders'.

One useful clinical indicator that the event was the trigger is that the intensity of the symptoms increases when the event is being recalled or recounted, and so symptoms wax and wane over time. There is also a presumption that without the stressor the disorder would not have arisen.

In ICD-10 (1), the duration of symptoms does not usually exceed 1 month (brief), and where it does, as a result of a continuing stressor or its consequences, it is coded as prolonged (F43.21). If the symptoms persist beyond 2 years, the diagnosis should be changed according to the clinical picture present, such as generalized anxiety, although the rationale for this 2-year threshold is unclear. The proposed criteria for ICD-11 (8, 14) also state that, ordinarily, symptoms will resolve within 6 months unless the consequences of the stressor continue. No time limits beyond that are mentioned and persisting symptoms will continue to be diagnosed as AD.

In DSM-5, resolution is defined as occurring no later than 6 months after the stressor or its consequences have ceased. No other time limits are mentioned.

Symptoms and impairment

Throughout the history of AD, specific constellations of symptoms have not been required and are not now required either in ICD-10 or DSM-5. In this, AD differs from most other disorders where there are operational definitions about the type, number, and duration of symptoms. Instead, AD is a diagnosis made on the basis of what is not present rather than what is, apart from the necessity for a prior stressor occurring within a set time before the onset of symptoms.

The only symptoms required are anxiety, depression, disturbance of conduct (including aggression), or combinations of these, and these are represented in the subtypes. The numbers of symptoms, or of those that co-occur, are not delineated as in other disorders.

ICD-10 required the presence of both symptoms and functional impairment (usually), while DSM required one or the other. This suggests that the threshold for making the diagnosis is higher in ICD-10. DSM-5 also requires that the symptoms should be clinically significant, although how this is evaluated is unclear and subject to criticism (15) (see also Chapter 3, p. 41).

Symptom profiles

Few studies have compared the symptom profiles of those with AD and those with depressive disorders. One that did so (16) only identified one symptom (viz., worry about physical health), which was more common in those with mild depressive episode than in those with either AD or moderately severe depressive episode. As numbers were small, this may have been due to a type II error.

One recent collaboration (Casey and Shevlin, pers. comm.) used latent class analysis to examine the symptom profiles—from the Inventory of Depressive Symptomatology (17)—of patients diagnosed clinically with either AD or depressive episode. Those with AD endorsed high frequency of mood reactivity and identified a particular quality to their mood. This was explored by the four statements from the item that tried to capture this, as listed in Box 6.1.

The more closely the quality of the mood resembles loss or bereavement (scores 0 and 1 in Box 6.1), the higher the endorsement by those with AD. Among those with AD there was low endorsement of 'leaden paralysis', psychomotor retardation, early morning wakening, hypersomnia, and somatic symptoms, while psychic anxiety was endorsed with moderate frequency. Questions about these symptoms might be of assistance in distinguishing AD from major depression/depressive episode in clinical practice.

ICD-11 (8, 14) now proposes specific criteria for ICD-11 that include preoccupation with the stressor and difficulty adapting, as evidenced by impaired concentration, sleep, low mood, and so on, and impairment in functioning (see also Chapter 1, pp. 7–8).

Box 6.1 Quality of mood question from the IDS-C (Inventory of Depressive Symptomatology, Clinician Rating)

0. Mood is normal or is virtually identical to feelings associated with bereavement or loss.

1. Mood is very much like sadness in bereavement or loss, although it may lack explanation, be associated with more anxiety, or be much more intense.

2. Less than half the time, mood is somewhat different from grief and it is difficult to explain to others.

3. Mood is almost always totally distinct from grief or loss.

Recent studies have focused on the proposed criteria for ICD-11 and have examined the symptoms of AD as proposed for it. Using a screening questionnaire, the Adjustment Disorder—New Module (ADNM) (18), investigators examined symptoms in those with a possible diagnosis of AD based on their responses to the questionnaire. It identified a six-factor model based on the 20 symptoms in the questionnaire, comprising avoidance, preoccupation, failure to adapt, depression, anxiety, and impulsivity. All were highly correlated, leading the authors to recommend a single dimension for AD, hence the decision to abandon the subtypes. In a further study, three latent classes emerged, representing mild, moderate, and severe forms of the condition (19). Since this work was carried out using the new concept of AD, it is unclear whether this symptom constellation is found in those whose diagnosis is based on the traditional concept of AD, as represented in ICD-10 and DSM-5, of which non-specific symptoms are the hallmark. This needs to be evaluated.

For now, the diagnostic criteria in DSM-5 and ICD-10 remain as before, with the focus being on the stressor and its close temporal relationship to the onset of general symptoms rather than on specific symptoms, apart from those of anxiety, depressed mood, and behavioural problems, as delineated in the subtypes.

Other elements in the presentation, not mentioned in the criteria, such as the ability to be distracted from one's sadness, the improvement in symptoms when the person is removed from the stressor by going on sick leave, and the absence of typical melancholic symptoms (e.g. diurnal mood swings, early morning wakening, or anhedonia) also point to a diagnosis of AD, provided of course there is a stressor that triggered the symptoms. The extent to which the symptoms appear to be driven by external factors (e.g. changing severity of the stressor in tandem with fluctuations in symptoms) also points to a possible AD, although the clinician must be cautious to avoid reinforcing faulty attributions as to causation. Sometimes this can only be fully assessed by watching and waiting or at other times by a trial of antidepressant medication, although the former should be the initial course of action if in doubt.

Collateral information about the timeline of symptoms in relation to the stressor, as well as details about past and family history, will also assist in making a diagnosis.

Differential diagnosis

The differential diagnosis in those suspected of having an AD is between a normal adaptive response on the one hand and a variety of overlapping conditions, either in evolution or fully developed as recognized syndromes, on the other.

Distinction from normal responses

The stress reaction has been recognized for decades, yet attempting to draw a line between what is normal and what crosses the line into disorder has challenged philosophical minds for centuries (see also Chapter 3, pp. 39–40).

The failure to differentiate appropriate, non-pathological reactions to stressful events from those that are pathological could lead to normal sadness being misdiagnosed as AD or depression (20) simply by the presence of symptoms. In the absence of criteria distinguishing normal from abnormal responses, clinical judgement at many levels

will play a prominent part in deciding whether the responses are pro-
portionate or excessive. These are listed in Box 6.2.

The diagnosis will have to take into account the personal
circumstances of the individual and the expression of symptoms
within the person's culture (see Box 6.2). For example, the loss of a job
for one person might be acceptable, while for another it could heap
poverty on a family. Cultural differences in the expression of emotion
will also need to be considered since some cultures are more expres-
sive than others. A knowledge of 'normal' coping with illness and
other stressful events is essential, and the diagnostic process will be
guided by the extent to which an individual's symptoms are in excess
of this, both in terms of severity and duration. For instance, failure to
appreciate that some societies grant compassionate leave from work
following bereavement might lead to such a person being identified as
disordered in another. Finally, the presence of functional impairment
is also an indicator of a pathological response.

With regard to symptoms, it is recommended that these should only
be regarded as excessive if they are 'clinically significant', although
this has not been defined and has been criticized as inadequate and
tautological (15, 21). One difficulty is that help-seeking—a likely determinant of clinical significance—varies between individuals, with
some seeking help at lower thresholds of symptoms and dysfunction
than others (see also Chapter 3, p. 41, for further discussion of this).
One possible definition is that symptoms should have resulted in
functional impairment in day-to-day activities. This is not a requirement of DSM-5, but it is in ICD-10.

Box 6.2 Distinguishing AD from normal responses to stressors

Personal circumstances and context of stressor
Proportionality between symptom severity and triggering event
Persistence beyond expected duration
Cultural norms for emotional response/expression
Duration and severity of functional impairment

Box 6.3 Vignette

A 40-year-old woman was told she was being made redundant from her work as an auctioneer 4 weeks ago. Since then, she cries many times every day, wondering how she is going to pay her mortgage (as a lone parent). She has trouble going to work because of her distress and has had 3 days on sick leave. She lies awake for several hours each night and has been prescribed hypnotics by her GP.

The person could be diagnosed with sub-syndromal symptomatic depression (any two or more simultaneous symptoms of depression, present for most or all of the time, at least 2 weeks in duration, associated with evidence of social dysfunction (25) or minor depression (not more than 4 symptoms for 2 weeks) or adjustment disorder (a subthreshold disorder in response to a stressful event) since the symptoms have arisen as a direct response to the stressor of being told she was being made redundant. AD would be the diagnosis if the focus was on the stressor.

Psychiatric disorders in evolution

The possibility that the symptoms represent a disorder in evolution, such as depressive episode or generalized anxiety disorder (GAD), should also be kept in mind since these too can be triggered by stressful events. However, the distorted perspective associated with these conditions can cause an incorrect attribution of causality to the event.

If the person has a prior history of depressive episode/major depression, the likelihood of the symptoms representing a disorder in evolution, rather than AD, should be considered. The symptom constellation might also represent an undertreated illness such as GAD or major depression/depressive episode.

These are also called 'subthreshold disorders', and various terms have been applied to them, including minor depression, sub-syndromal symptomatic depression, and subclinical depression (22), to mention but a few. The terminology is confusing. Their importance lies in the incapacity associated with them—hence the importance of identifying and offering treatment (23), and the possibility that some may develop into a full-threshold depressive episode. These are discussed further in Chapter 3, pp. 46–7.

The relevance of this heterogeneous terminology to AD is that it is possible to simultaneously meet the diagnostic criteria for both AD and one or more of the subthreshold conditions listed above (24), depending on whether the emphasis is on the symptoms or on the stressor. However, the course of AD differs from that of the other subthreshold disorders and the interventions are also likely to differ. One simple strategy for distinguishing AD from these other disorders is to adopt a 'watch and wait approach' rather than rushing to intervene in what may be a self-limiting condition requiring only minimal or brief interventions.

The following example illustrates the similarity between AD and subthreshold depressive disorders.

Depressive episode/major depression

This is one of the conditions with which AD is most likely to be conflated. There is a symptom overlap, and according to ICD-10 and DSM-5, once the required numbers of symptoms are present for more than 2 weeks, the diagnosis changes from AD to major depression even where there is a clear relationship between the occurrence of a stressor and the onset of symptoms and AD might clinically seem the more appropriate diagnosis. This is particularly so in DSM-5, where the symptoms are much more tightly delineated than in ICD-10. If the new criteria are accepted for ICD-11, this problem will no longer exist, as AD will be a full-threshold disorder that can be diagnosed at any point once a stressor is present. The diagnosis will thus be based on clinical judgement concerning symptoms based on the totality of the person's history rather than the exclusively symptom-based approach currently used.

A useful guide is that the symptoms are not as pervasive in AD and the person will describe some improvement when physically or cognitively remote from the situation. For example, a person being bullied at work who takes time off will experience a reduction in symptoms when away from the workplace but may become upset when speaking about it or when in physical proximity to it.

Generalized anxiety disorder

Generalized anxiety disorder (GAD) also overlaps with AD, of anxiety subtype. There is very little to assist the clinician in distinguishing one from the other since GAD is also often triggered by a stressor. As with depressive episodes above, symptoms are likely to be worse in either cognitive or physical proximity to the stressor or its consequences. This requires further study.

PTSD and acute stress disorder

In ICD-10, the only symptom differences between PTSD and acute stress disorder (ASD) are in their time of onset relative to the stressor. ASD has symptoms similar to PTSD but they are present in ASD from 1 week after the event to up to 6 weeks after it, and if they continue beyond that cut-off they are then labelled as PTSD: thus one merges into the other. Both require extreme stressors.

There is a question as to whether AD arises after exposure to life-threatening/traumatic events, or whether ASD/PTSD is always the outcome. AD can occur in situations that might potentially cause ASD/PTSD, and it cannot be assumed that PTSD is the inevitable result of such exposure. DSM-IV recognized this and allowed for subthreshold PTSD to be classified as AD, but this has now changed as DSM-5 has incorporated a PTSD-like syndrome into its classification when the full criteria for a trauma and stressor-related disorder are not met. This is called 'unspecified trauma and stressor-related disorder'. Recent evidence supports the view that traumatic stressors can cause outcomes other than PTSD. One study carried out in areas of high conflict where ordinarily PTSD might be expected to be the result identified AD as one outcome, ranging in incidence from 5.7% to 40% (13), and this study based the diagnosis of AD on the new concept: thus, ICD-11 is likely to allow for a diagnosis of AD even in circumstances where the stressor was such that it could also cause PTSD.

ICD-10 excludes events that are unusual or catastrophic, but in clinical practice, when symptoms not amounting to PTSD/ASD are present, they are diagnosed as AD. It is unclear how ICD-11 will deal with subthreshold PTSD/ASD.

Dysthymia

For those experiencing long-standing stressors or their consequences, the persistently low mood that results may be misclassified as dysthymia, or even as enduring personality change after psychiatric illness (ICD only) or depressive personality disorder (DSM only).

Comorbidity

In the current classifications, there is no possibility of comorbidity, since AD cannot be diagnosed in the presence of another threshold condition. The low mood associated with substance misuse and with personality disorder, especially emotionally unstable personality disorder (EUPD), should not be misdiagnosed as AD, and so the two cannot be said to be comorbid. In the case of substance misuse the depressogenic effects of alcohol and other substances may be mistaken for AD if there are concurrent stressors in the person's life. In those with EUPD, the rapid emotional shifts that often occur in response to minor stressors should not be diagnosed as AD as these are an inherent part of EUPD.

Conclusions

AD is a challenge to diagnose in clinical settings partly because it is often not considered except in the emergency department after an episode of self-harm. The possibility that what seems to be AD might be another developing disorder or an undertreated one needs to be considered. AD should not be diagnosed in those with rapidly shifting moods due to EUPD or depressive substances. There is an emerging pattern of symptoms from recent research that might help distinguish AD from major depression/DE, and other symptoms, more closely resembling PTSD, have now been suggested for ICD-11. The validity of these as indicative of AD, as currently diagnosed and understood, needs to be tested.

References

1. **World Health Organization**. International classification of diseases. 10th ed. Geneva: World Health Organization; 1994.
2. **American Psychiatric Association**. Diagnostic and statistical manual of mental disorders. 5th ed. Washington, DC: American Psychiatric Association; 2013.

3. McHugh PR, Slavney PR. Mental illness—comprehensive evaluation or checklist? N Engl J Med. 2012;**366**:1853–5.

4. Taggart C, O'Grady J, Stevenson M, Hand E, McClelland R, Kelly C. Accuracy of diagnosis and routine psychiatric assessment in patients presenting to an accident and emergency department. Gen Hosp Psychiatry. 2006;**8**:330–5.

5. For-Wey L, Lee F-Y, Shu B-C. The premorbid personality in military students with adjustment disorder. Mil Psychol. 2006;**18**(1):77–88.

6. Doherty AM, Jabbar F, Kelly BD, Casey P. Distinguishing between adjustment disorder and depressive episode in clinical practice: the role of personality disorder. J Affect Disord. 2014;**168**:78–85.

7. Na K-S, Oh S-J, Jung H-Y, Lee SI, Kim Y-K, Han C, et al. Temperament and character of young male conscripts with adjustment disorder: a case-control study. J Nerv Ment Dis. 2012;**200**(11):973–7.

8. Maercker A, Einsle F, Kollner V. Adjustment disorders as stress response syndromes: a new diagnostic concept and its exploration in a medical sample. Psychopathology. 2007;**40**(3):135–46.

9. Despland JN, Monod L, Ferrero F. Clinical relevance of adjustment disorder in DSM-III-R and DSM-IV. Compr Psychiatry. 1995;**36**(6):454–60.

10. O'Donnell ML, Alkemade N, Creamer M, McFarlane AC, Silove D, Bryant RA, et al. A longitudinal study of adjustment disorder after trauma exposure. Am J Psychiatry. 2016;**173**(12):1231–8.

11. American Psychiatric Association. Diagnostic and statistical manual of mental disorders. 4th ed. Washington, DC: American Psychiatric Association; 1994.

12. American Psychiatric Association. Diagnostic and statistical manual of mental disorders. 4th ed, text revision. Washington, DC: American Psychiatric Association; 2000.

13. Dobricki M, Komproe IH, de Jong JTVM, Maercker A. Adjustment disorders after severe life-events in four post-conflict settings. Soc Psychiatry Psychiatr Epidemiol. 2010;**45**(1):39–46.

14. Maercker A, Brewin C, Bryant RA, Cloitre M, Reed GM, van Ommeren M, et al. Proposals for mental disorders specifically associated with stress in the International Classification of Diseases-11. Lancet. 2013;**381**:1683–5.

15. Frances A. Problems in defining clinical significance in epidemiological studies. Arch Gen Psychiatry. 1998;**55**(2):119.

16. Casey P, Maracy M, Kelly BD, Lehtinen V, Ayuso-Mateos JL, Dalgard OS, et al. Can adjustment disorder and depressive episode be distinguished? Results from ODIN. J Affect Disord. 2006;**92**(2–3):291–7.

17. Trivedi MH, Rush AJ, Ibrahim HM, Carmody TJ, Biggs MM, Suppes T, et al. The Inventory of Depressive Symptomatology, Clinician Rating (IDS-C) and Self-Report (IDS-SR), and the Quick Inventory of Depressive

Symptomatology, Clinician Rating (QIDS-C) and Self-Report (QIDS-SR) in public sector patients with mood disorders: a psychometric evaluation. Psychol Med. 2004;**34**:73–82.

18. Einsle F, Köllner V, Dannemann S, Maercker A. Development and validation of a self-report for the assessment of adjustment disorders. Psychol Health Med. 2010;**15**(5):584–95.

19. Glaesmer H, Romppel M, Brähler E, Hinz A, Maercker A. Adjustment disorder as proposed for ICD-11: dimensionality and symptom differentiation. Psychiatry Res. 2015;**229**(3):940–8.

20. Horwitz AV, Wakefield JC. The loss of sadness: How psychiatry transformed normal sorrow into depressive disorder. New York: NY Oxford University Press; 2007.

21. Spitzer RL, Wakefield JC. DSM-IV diagnostic criterion for clinical significance: does it help solve the false positives problem? Am J Psychiatry. 1999;**156**:1856–64.

22. Rodriguez MR, Nuevo R, Chatterji S, Ayuso-Matoes JL. Definitions and factors associated with subthreshold depressive conditions: a systematic review. BMC Psychiatry. 2012;**12**:181.

23. Fogel J, Eaton WW, Ford DE. Minor depression as a predictor of the first onset of major depressive disorder over a 15-year follow-up. Acta Psychiatr Scand. 2006;**113**(1):36–43.

24. Takei N, Sugihara G. Diagnostic ambiguity of subthreshold depression: minor depression vs. adjustment disorder with depressive mood. Acta Psychiatr Scand. 2006;**114**(2):144.

25. Judd LL, Rapaport MH, Paulus MP, Brown JL. Subsyndromal symptomatic depression: a new mood disorder? J Clin Psychiatry. 1994;**55**(April suppl):18–28.

Chapter 7

Treatment of adjustment disorders

Patricia Casey

The approach to treatment for those with AD is under-researched, although it is suggested that in many, no treatment may be required, as these are self-limiting conditions and when treatment is required it should be brief and psychological (1). Others argue that treatment hastens recovery and thus alleviates suffering, particularly as they are common and may be protracted if the stressor continues, resulting in a substantial decline in quality of life, persistent distress, and suicidal behaviour (2, 3). Older recommendations based on Expert Consensus (4) recommended psychological and pharmacological interventions, particularly benzodiazepines, although for those at risk of dependence or who had alcohol dependence, buspirone or tricyclic antidepressants were considered as alternatives.

The therapeutic focus in recent years has almost exclusively been on brief psychological interventions (1). The National Institute for Health and Care Excellence (NICE) does not provide guidelines on the treatment of AD. One reason for this may be that few randomized controlled trials (RTCs) have been conducted, particularly for pharmacological interventions. There are a number of reasons for this, including the following:

1. AD is usually a transient condition and may have resolved before the trial is completed

2. There are no specific diagnostic criteria, so obtaining homogeneous groups of patients is problematic

3. The absence of specific criteria compromises the monitoring of symptoms or functioning when examining the outcome of an intervention

4. The symptoms may have resolved before the onset of action of medication, e.g., antidepressants or psychological therapies

5. Questions about the timing of the outcome assessment, e.g., should this happen when the stressor has stabilized or has terminated, or at an agreed time point post intervention?

6. The stressor attributes add a further confound to obtaining a homogeneous sample because of the differences in the nature (quality), severity (quantity), and acuteness (less than 6 months) or chronicity (more than 6 months) of the stressors.

Despite these impediments there have been some studies of psychotherapy, of herbal remedies, and of eye movement desensitization and reprocessing, but very few studies of pharmacological therapies.

The absence of studies of pharmacotherapy is a serious lacuna, since despite recommendations that psychological therapies are to be preferred, and the absence of evidence for the benefits of antidepressants, the latter are now the most commonly prescribed medications in the United States (5), with the proportion in the general population receiving them almost doubling from 5.84% in 1996 to 10.12% in 2005. Numerically, this represents an increase from 13 million to 27 million persons on antidepressants. Their use in AD shows the greatest increase among those with common mental disorders, from a rate of 22.26% in 1996 to 39.37% in 2005.

Psychotherapy: general principles

Traditionally, when treating AD, most experts recommend integrating elements from psychosocial treatments which are established and effective for other psychiatric disorders (6). This presumes that the mechanisms of change from those treatments can be transferred to AD.

The goal of treatment in AD is to reduce the impact of the stressor, reduce the symptoms that have resulted, enhance the individual's ability to cope with stressors that cannot be reduced or removed, and establish a support system to maximize adaptation.

The first step is to note significant dysfunction caused by the stressor and to help the patient moderate this. Many stressors (e.g., those resulting from taking on more responsibility than can be managed by the individual) can be avoided or minimized, while others cannot be avoided yet may generate an excessive reaction by the patient. These may include withdrawing from one's social activities or engaging in self-harm or suicide attempts. The role of the therapist is to assist the patient in verbalizing his/her distress and emotions rather than turning these into destructive actions. The meaning of the stressor for the patient needs to be elucidated. For example, moving from a long-standing family home may represent a severing of ties with a happy past for an uncertain future. If this is seen as an end rather than a new beginning, it may have a devastating effect on the patient's emotions and functioning.

A myriad of therapies have been used. These range from supportive psychotherapy (7), cognitive-behavioural therapy (CBT) (8), interpersonal psychotherapy (9), client-centred psychotherapy (10), Gestalt psychotherapy (11), and psychodynamic interventions (7, 12), to third-wave CBT techniques such as meditation (13). When the concerns and conflicts that the patient is experiencing have been considered, the next step is to identify strategies to reduce the stressors, enhance the patient's coping skills, help the patient gain perspective on the adversity, and establish relationships (e.g., a support network) to assist in the management of the stressors and the self. Despite trials of these therapies, there are methodological problems since some are not randomized (9) and others have small sample sizes (7, 13).

All the above therapies have been used in a variety of psychiatric disorders, and it is assumed that their mechanism of action will also transfer to AD. In general, the quality of the studies on these therapies is limited, and in some cases it is unclear whether the recipients have AD since many are reported as having depressive symptoms rather than meeting criteria for a specific diagnosis (7). Some of these therapies will be discussed in further detail below.

Interpersonal psychotherapy

Interpersonal psychotherapy was applied to depressed HIV-positive outpatients and found to be effective, although the study was an open-label pilot study with a sample size of 22 subjects receiving therapy over 16 sessions (9). The focus was on psycho-education, formulation of problems from an interpersonal perspective, and identification of the interpersonal areas of problems such as grief, role changes, and so on.

Brief therapies

Those with AD benefit most from brief psychotherapy by reframing the meaning of the stressor(s) (14). However, multiple or ongoing stressors along with the personality of the individual may compromise this, and lengthier interventions may be required. In the context of military psychiatry, where AD is particularly common, some have emphasized the treatment variables of Brevity, Immediacy, Centrality, Expectance, Proximity, and Simplicity (the 'BICEPS' principles). The treatment approach is brief—usually no more than 72 hours (15).

Some studies have examined an array of depressive and anxiety disorders and included ADs in their cohorts. A recent trial comparing brief dynamic therapy with brief supportive therapy in 30 patients with minor depressive disorders, including ADs, found that while both therapies proved efficacious in reducing symptoms, brief dynamic therapy was more effective at 6-month follow up (7). The results for those with AD were not analyzed separately.

Support groups

Support groups have been used to assist some patients with life-threatening illness, particularly those with cancer, but the studies in question do not specifically deal with AD but select those who are 'distressed' or 'depressed' (16). While benefits in relation to coping, distress, and quality of life have been identified (17), there is an absence of evidence of their benefit to those with AD.

Resilience building

There is an increasing emphasis on resilience in psychiatry, both as an attribute that protects against certain mental illnesses in the face of trauma and stress such as PTSD (post-traumatic stress disorder) or AD, but also as something to be harnessed in treating these conditions and thus preventing further occurrences in the face of re-traumatization.

While there have been no specific studies on AD, the conceptual closeness between it and PTSD suggests that resilience-enhancing techniques might have a role in treating ADs. Southwick & Charney (18) state that 'resilience is generally understood as the ability to bounce back from hardship and trauma', and they emphasize that people's reactions to stress differ remarkably. The manner in which individuals respond to stress 'depends on numerous genetic, developmental, cognitive, psychological, and neurobiological risk and protective factors'. The psychosocial variables associated with resilience, according to this research, include optimism, cognitive flexibility, active coping skills, maintaining a supportive social environment, attending to one's physical wellbeing, and having a personal moral compass that shows the individual understands their purpose and meaning in the world. This may include harnessing spiritual and religious values.

One such study (19) offered a brief resilience-building intervention to over 1,600 soldiers returning from combat in Iraq deemed to be at high risk of PTSD, mood disorders, and other 'transition problems'. It showed that those receiving the intervention showed better adjustment across the range of mental health disorders being studied than the control group. One problem with this study is that it focused on symptoms rather than specific diagnoses, so there is no certainty that this intervention is beneficial specifically in AD; but as this is the most common diagnosis in the military it is a possible conclusion. Clearly, further studies specifically in those with AD are necessary.

Specific therapies for AD

Therapies specific to AD are currently being developed and tested. One such example is the TAPS (Treatment for Anxiety and Physical Symptoms) programme, a problem-solving approach for individuals and groups (20). In a pilot study, the programme achieved a significant decrease in anxiety and anger symptoms, and an improvement in mood, as compared to a waiting-list control group. A second intervention developed to treat AD symptoms employs a virtual-reality self-help programme named 'EMMA's world', which is used as an addition to face-to-face treatment (21). This programme aims to enable activation and processing of emotions and cognitions based on the theory that with repeated exposure, fear habituates.

Low-threshold interventions are likely to be more appropriate for AD patients than longer interventions, and this has been recognized for decades. These include self-help measures, such as biblio-therapy or online therapy, as a cost-efficient alternative to face-to-face psycho-therapy. A self-help manual and a pilot e-version specifically based on the ICD-11 conceptualization are currently being evaluated (22, 23). These approaches are in line with the stepped-care model and are providing the first line in resolving symptoms. Thereafter, face-to-face therapy can be instituted if required (24).

These are new therapies. Further studies using appropriate sample sizes are required before they can become accepted as having benefit and as disorder-specific interventions.

Mirror therapy

Mirror therapy was originally developed for those with phantom limb pain. It involves the use of a mirror which assists the patient in configuring a new body map as a consequence of the visual feedback. It has been adapted by some (11) for use in those with low mood or 'psychological pain' following acute myocardial infarction. The study involved 122 subjects aged 30–60 years and was compared with Gestalt therapy, medical conversations, and a control group. As part of the treatment, a mirror is used to encourage patient acceptance of his/her physical limitations that resulted from the lack of past self-care behaviours. Depressive symptoms improved in all treatment groups compared with the control sample, but mirror therapy was significantly more effective than other treatments in decreasing symptoms of AD at 6-month follow up.

Eye movement desensitization and reprocessing

The first intervention study which considered the conceptual closeness of AD and PTSD was eye movement desensitization and reprocessing (EMDR). Already in use in those with PTSD, the author studied its use in nine patients with AD (25). The results demonstrated significant improvement among those with anxious or mixed features, but not among those with depressed mood; those with ongoing stressors did not demonstrate improvement. Clearly, further studies are required if this is to be recommended for use in this group of patients. Another study (26) examined 90 subjects exposed to distressing events and not meeting criteria for PTSD. Subjects were randomized to EMDR, active listening, or waiting-list control. Their levels of anxiety were significantly lower after recall of the event, and their overall score in the Impact of Events Scale was significantly lower than in the comparison groups.

Herbal and alternative remedies

Most double blind RTCs in AD have used herbal remedies. These have mainly focused on the AD with anxiety (ADWA) subtype. The mode of action of such remedies is unclear.

One 25-week, multicentre, double-blind RTC involved 101 outpatients with a variety of anxiety disorders including ADWA. It compared placebo with kava-kava. The latter was reported to be effective in ADWA in comparison with placebo and did not produce side effects (27). Another RTC (28) assigned 91 patients with ADWA to receive either Euphytose—a preparation containing a combination of plant extracts (*Crataegus, Ballota, Passiflora,* and *Valeriana,* which have mild sedative effects, and *Cola* and *Paullinia,* which mainly act as mild stimulants)—or placebo for 28 days. Patients taking the experimental drugs improved significantly more than those taking placebo. A further study compared *Ginkgo biloba* with placebo (29) on 107 patients with generalized anxiety disorder (GAD, n = 82) or ADWA (n = 25). The trial lasted 4 weeks and intention-to-treat analysis was used. Both high- and low-dose *Ginkgo biloba* was associated with a significant improvement in anxiety and in several secondary measures in the total sample and in the ADWA group, although the small number in the latter group did not allow for statistical analysis.

There is also some evidence that, for AD with anxiety and depression, yoga might be beneficial (13). In a controlled study comparing meditation with group counselling for 24 weeks, in a sample of 30 subjects, measures of mean scores at 28 weeks between experimental and control groups were significantly different in favour of the experimental group, and pre- and post-intervention comparisons were also favourable for the experimental group on a number of scales.

Two mindfulness studies deserve consideration. One examined the impact of mindfulness training in a diagnostically heterogeneous group of psychiatric outpatients (30). The study involved 143 patients, including 14 with AD, and the remainder had depressive illness, bipolar disorder, and anxiety. Training consisted of eight 2½-hour sessions. Those with AD showed a positive response on all outcome measures, as did the other groups, with the exception of those with bipolar disorder, where the effect size for some measures was lower. Mindfulness group therapy was compared with individual CBT in an 8-week non-inferiority study of 215 patients with common mental disorders (including AD) in primary care. For both interventions the scores decreased significantly and there was no difference between them (31).

Application of psychotherapy in special groups and settings

Occupational intervention; a CBT approach combined with problem-solving treatment

Occupational settings are rife with mental health problems and especially AD. They are often described in general practitioners' notes as 'work-related stress'. Absenteeism rates are high and this sometimes results in early retirement. The goal of achieving early return to work is difficult to achieve, but is the aspiration of governments around the world (see also Chapter 11). Thus, treatments to improve on absenteeism rates are keenly sought after.

A Cochrane systematic review (32) examined either CBT or problem-solving therapy (PST) to facilitate a return to work in those with AD. Nine out of 59 studies met the inclusion criteria, and involved 1,546 participants. Seven of the nine studies were carried out in the Netherlands—one in Denmark and one in Sweden. No RCTs were found of pharmacological interventions, exercise programmes, or employee assistance programmes. Even the nine studies selected had the major problem of heterogeneity of psychiatric diagnosis. 'Burn out', 'stress', 'neurasthenia', 'work-related stress', and 'minor mental disorder' were considered as diagnoses of AD in several studies. Some studies were included if as few as 30% of the diagnoses were 'pure' AD. Finally, AD was diagnosed using varied criteria, screening instruments, and diagnosticians. The review found that although CBT was superior to placebo, it did not reduce the number of days to either partial or full-time return to work when compared to no treatment. Problem-solving therapy, however, reduced the time to partial return to work compared to non-guideline-based care, while it did not influence the number of days to full-time return when followed for 1–2 years.

One of the studies included in the review used an 'activating intervention' for ADs (33). In this study, 192 employees were randomized to receive either the intervention or usual care. The intervention consisted of an individual cognitive-behavioural approach to a graded activity, similar to stress-inoculation training. The worker was asked to do more demanding and complicated activities as treatment progressed. Goals of treatment emphasized the acquisition of coping skills and the regaining of control.

The treatment proved to be effective in decreasing sick leave duration and shortening long-term absenteeism when compared with the control cohort. Ultimately, it formed the basis for the 'Dutch Practice Guidelines for the Treatment of ADs in Primary and Occupational Health Care', prepared by 21 occupational health physicians and one psychologist, and subsequently reviewed and tested by 15 experts, including several psychiatrists, and psychologists, and 21 practising occupational health physicians.

Other studies on return-to-work interventions focus on common mental disorders, including AD, but without any subgroup analysis to specifically evaluate those with AD.

Psychotherapeutic interventions for the elderly

Elderly patients are particularly vulnerable to the development of ADs as the stress of interpersonal losses, medical illness, and multiple medications abound. Life transitions such as relocating to a nursing home or losing one's driving privileges are commonly experienced as stressors in the elderly. Any treatment that strengthens a patient's ego by helping him/her acknowledge the stressor and by promoting effective coping strategies is useful in this population. An active therapeutic stance and the use of life review foster a sense of mastery over the stressor (34).

Pharmacotherapy

Although psychotherapy is the mainstay of treatment for the ADs, there is data, described above, to show that antidepressants are prescribed for this condition despite the limited evidence to support their use (5). Strain et al. (35) observed that AD patients seen in psychiatric consultation in the general hospital setting were equally as likely to receive medication as were patients with major psychiatric disorders, despite a paucity of evidence to support this. One of the first studies on AD (subtype unspecified), which compared placebo, supportive psychotherapy, an antidepressant, and a benzodiazepine, found no difference between any intervention and all patients improved (36). A double-blind study in primary care in those with ADWA (37) found that tianeptine, alprazolam, and mianserin were equally effective. Among general-practice patients with AD, etifoxine and lorazepam were compared in a double-blind study involving almost 200 patients. Both agents led to a significant reduction in symptoms, but etifoxine was associated with a larger number of participants improving markedly and fewer developing rebound anxiety on withdrawal of the medication (38). Treatment was evaluated over 28 days. In a further study in those with ADWA, etifoxine, a non-benzodiazepine anxiolytic, was shown to be superior to alprazolam in an RTC of over 200 subjects in primary care (39). Two pilot studies of cancer patients (40) and of HIV-positive patients (41) compared trazodone with clorazepate and found the antidepressant superior to the benzodiazepine.

One study conducted in primary care (42) suggested a benefit from antidepressants in those with AD with depressed mood seen in primary care. The results indicated that neither those with major depression nor those with AD demonstrated a difference in clinical response to any particular antidepressant. Those with a diagnosis of AD, however, were twice as likely to respond to standard antidepressant treatment as those with major depression. On the surface, this study suggests that antidepressants are effective in treating AD with depressed mood in the primary care setting, but this was a retrospective case-note evaluation and so it has very limited implications concerning the use of antidepressants in this group.

Because RTCs examining AD seem rare, a Cochrane meta-analysis is under way to evaluate the psychopharmacological treatment of ADs. This is an important investigation as few RCTs have focused on pharmacological treatment in AD (43). The protocol has been published, but definitive results are not yet available.

Conclusion

There is uncertainty as to the appropriate interventions, if any, for those with AD. There are few RTCs of either psychological or pharmacological interventions. Given the high prevalence of AD in certain clinical settings, such as liaison psychiatry, and in occupational settings, especially the military, effective disorder-specific interventions should be developed and evaluated. Low-threshold, non-invasive intervention such as self-help, monitoring, and psycho-education may be appropriate for AD. The explicit stress-response model proposed for ICD-11 suggests that the effectiveness of PTSD-specific interventions such as imaginary exposure or EMDR should also be investigated in the treatment of AD. However, because AD is generally self-resolving, selecting the control intervention will be important in order to establish whether any specific treatment is required or whether general supportive measures are all that is required. Among the pharmacological treatments, etifoxine has been shown in a few trials to be superior to other agents. There is an absence of evidence regarding the benefit of antidepressants. Herbal remedies have been shown to be effective in some studies, but their mode of action is unclear.

References

1. **Strain J, Friedman MJ.** Adjustment disorders. In: Gabbard GO, editor. Gabbard's treatments of psychiatric disorders. 5th ed. Arlington, VA: American Psychiatric Publishing; 2015. p. 519–29.

2. **Gradus JL, Qin P, Lincoln AK, Miller M, Lawler E, Lash TL.** The association between adjustment disorder diagnosed at psychiatric treatment facilities and completed suicide. Clin Epidemiol. 2010;**2**:23–8.

3. **Casey P, Jabbar F, O'Leary E, Doherty AM.** Suicidal behaviours in adjustment disorder and depressive episode. J Affect Disord. 2015;**174**:441–6.

4. **Uhlenhuth EH, Balter MB, Ban TA, Yang K.** International study of expert judgement on therapeutic use of benzodiazepines and other psychotherapeutic medications: II. Pharmacotherapy of anxiety disorders. J Affect Disord. 1995;**35**(4):153–62.

5. **Olfson M, Marcus SC.** National patterns in antidepressant medication treatment. Arch Gen Psychiatry. 2009;(66)**8**:848–56.

6. **O'Connor BP, Cartwright H.** Adjustment disorder. In: Sturmey P, Hersen M, editors. Handbook of evidence-based practice in clinical psychology. Hoboken, NJ: John Wiley; 2012. p. 493–506.

7. **Maina G, Forner F, Bogetto F.** Randomized controlled trial comparing brief dynamic and supportive therapy with waiting list condition in minor depressive disorders. Psychother Psychosom. 2005;**74**:43–50.

8. **Dalgaard L, Eskildsen A, Carstensen O, Willert MV, Andersen JH, Glasscock DJ.** Changes in self-reported sleep and cognitive failures: a randomized controlled trial of a stress management intervention. Scand J Work Environ Health. 2014;**40**(6):569–81.

9. **Markowitz JC, Klerman GL, Perry SW.** Interpersonal psychotherapy of depressed HIV-positive outpatients. Hosp Community Psychiatry. 1992;**43**(9):885–90.

10. **Altenhöfer A, Schulz W, Schwab R, Eckert J.** Psychotherapie von Anpassungsstörungen. Ist eine auf 12 Sitzungen begrenzte Gesprächspsychotherapie ausreichend wirksam? [Is psychotherapy if limited to 12 sessions sufficiently effective?]. Psychotherapeut. 2007;**52**(1):24–34.

11. **González-Jaimes EI, Turnbull-Plaza B.** Selection of psychotherapeutic treatment for adjustment disorder with depressive mood due to acute myocardial infarction. Arch Med Res. 2003;**34**(4):298–304.

12. **Ben-Itzhak S, Bluvstein I, Schreiber S, Aharonov-Zaig I, Maor M, Lipnik R, et al.** The effectiveness of brief versus intermediate duration psychodynamic psychotherapy in the treatment of adjustment disorder. J Contemp Psychother. 2012;**42**(4):249–56.

13. **Srivastava M, Talukdar U, Lahan V.** Meditation for the management of adjustment disorder anxiety and depression. Complement Ther Clin Pract. 2011;**17**(4):241–5.

14. **Sifneos PE.** Brief dynamic and crisis therapy. In: Comprehensive textbook psychiatry IV. 5th ed, vol **2. Kaplan HI,** Sadock BJ, editors. Baltimore, MD: Williams & Wilkins; 1989. p. 1562–7.

15. **True PK, Benway MW.** Treatment of stress reaction prior to combat using the 'BICEPS' model. Mil Med. 1992;**157**:380–1.

16. **Fawzy FI, Canada AL, Fawzy NW.** Malignant melanoma: effects of a brief, structured psychiatric intervention on survival and recurrence at 10-year follow-up. Arch Gen Psychiatry. 2003;**60**:100–10.

17. **Spiegel D.** Mind matters in cancer survival. JAMA. 2011;**305**:502–3.

18. **Southwick SM, Charney DS.** The science of resilience: implications for the prevention and treatment of depression. Science. 2012;**338**:79–82.

19. **Castro CA, Adler AB, McGurk, Bliese PD.** Mental health training with soldiers four months after returning from Iraq: randomization by platoon. J Trauma Stress. 2012;**25**:376–83.

20. **Reschke K, Teichmann K.** Entwicklung und Evaluation eines kognitiv-behavioralen Therapieprogramms für Patienten mit Anpassungsstörung [Development and evaluation of a cognitive-behavioral psychotherapy program for patients with adjustment disorder]. Psychosom und Kons. 2008;**2**(2):98–103.

21. **Andreu-Mateu S, Botella C, Quero S, Guillén V, Baños R.** La utilización de la realidad virtual y estrategias de psicología positiva en el tratamiento de los trastornos adaptativos [The use of virtual reality and positive psychology strategies for the treatment of adjustment disorders]. Behav Psychol Conduct. 2012;**20**:323–48.

22. **Bachem R.** Self-help interventions for adjustment disorder problems: a randomized waiting-list controlled study in a sample of burglary victims. Cogn Behav Ther. 2016;**45**(5):397–413.

23. **Maercker A, Bachem R, Lorenz L, Moser CT, Berger T.** Adjustment disorders are uniquely suited for eHealth interventions: concept and case study. JMIR Ment Health. 2015;**2**(2):e15.

24. **Williams C, Martinez R.** Increasing access to CBT: stepped care and CBT self-help models in practice. Behav Cogn Psychother. 2008;**36**(6): 675–83.

25. **Mihelich ML.** Eye movement desensitization and reprocessing treatment of adjustment disorder. Diss Abstr Int. 2000;**61**:1091.

26. **Cvetek R.** EMDR treatment of distressful experiences that fail to meet the criteria for PTSD. J EMDR Pract Res. 2008;**2**(1):2–14.

27. **Voltz HP, Kieser M.** Kava-kava extract WS 1490 versus placebo in anxiety disorders: a randomised placebo-controlled 25-week outpatient trial. Pharmacopsychiatry. 1997;**30**:1–5.

28. **Bourin M, Bougerol T, Guitton B, Broutin E.** A combination of plant extracts in the treatment of outpatients with adjustment disorder and anxious mood: controlled study versus placebo. Fundam Clin Pharmacol 1994;**11**:127–32.

29. **Woelk H, Arnoldt KH, Kieser M, Hoerr R.** Ginkgo biloba special extract EGb 761 in generalized anxiety disorder and adjustment disorder with anxious mood: a randomized, double-blind, placebo-controlled trial. J Psychiatr Res. 2007;**41**(6):472–80.

30. **Bos EH, Merea R, van den Brink E, Sanderman R, Bartels-Velthuis AA.** Mindfulness training in a heterogeneous psychiatric sample: outcome evaluation and comparison of different diagnostic groups. J Clin Psychol. 2014;**70**(1):60–71.

31. **Sundquist J, Lilja Å, Palmér K, Memon AA, Wang X, Johansson LM, et al.** Mindfulness group therapy in primary care patients with depression, anxiety and stress and adjustment disorders: randomised controlled trial. Br J Psychiatry. 2015;**206**(2):128–35.

32. **Arends I, Bruinvels DJ, Rebergen DS, Nieuwenhuijsen K, Madan I, Neumeyer-Gromen A, et al.** Interventions to facilitate return to work in adults with adjustment disorders. Cochrane Database Syst Rev. 2012; Issue 12. Art. No.: CD006389. DOI: 10.1002/14651858.CD006389.pub2

33. **van der Klink JJ, Blonk RW, Schene AH, van Dijk FJ.** Reducing long term sickness absence by an activating intervention in adjustment

disorders: a cluster randomised controlled design. Occup Environ Med. 2003;**60**(6):429–37.

34. **Frankel M.** Ego enhancing treatment for adjustment disorders of later life. J Geriatr Psychiatry. 2001;**34**:221–3.

35. **Strain JJ, Smith GC, Hammer JS.** Adjustment disorder: a multisite study of its utilisation and interventions in the consultation-liaison psychiatry setting. Gen Hosp Psychiatry. 1998;**20**(3):139–49.

36. **De Leo D.** Treatment of adjustment disorders: a comparative evaluation. Psychol Rep. 1989;**64**(1):51–4.

37. **Ansseau M, Bataille M, Briole G, de Nayer A, Fauchère PA, Ferrero F,** et al. Controlled comparison of tianeptine, alprazolam and mianserin in the treatment of adjustment disorders with anxiety and depression. Hum Psychopharmacol. 1996;**11**:293–98.

38. **Nguyen N, Fakra E, Pradel V, Jouve E, Alquier C, Le Guern ME,** et al. Efficacy of etifoxine compared to lorazepam monotherapy in the treatment of patients with adjustment disorders with anxiety: a double-blind controlled study in general practice. Hum Psychopharmacol. 2006;**21**(3):139–49.

39. **Stein DJ.** Etifoxine versus alprazolam for the treatment of adjustment disorder with anxiety: a randomized controlled trial. Adv Ther. 2015;**32**(1):57–68.

40. **Razavi D, Kormoss N, Collard A, Farvacques C, Delvaux N.** Comparative study of the efficacy and safety of trazadone versus clorazepate in the treatment of adjustment disorders in cancer patients: a pilot study. J Int Med Res. 1999;**27**:264–72.

41. **De Wit S, Cremers L, Hirsch D, Zulian C, Clumeck N, Kormoss N.** Efficacy and safety of trazodone versus clorazepate in the treatment of HIV-positive subjects with adjustment disorders: a pilot study. J Int Med Res. 1999;**27**(5):223–32.

42. **Hameed, U, Schwartz, TL, Malhotra K, West RL, Bertone F.** Antidepressant treatment in the primary care office: outcomes for adjustment disorder versus major depression. Ann Clin Psychiatry. 2005;**17**(2):77–81.

43. **Casey P, Pillay D, Wilson L, Maercker A, Rice A, Kelly B.** Pharmacological interventions for adjustment disorders in adults (Protocol). Cochrane Database Syst Rev. 2013; Issue 6. Art. No.: CD010530. DOI: 10.1002/ 14651858.CD010530

Chapter 8

The course and prognosis of adjustment disorders

Patricia Casey

The DSM-5 (*Diagnostic and Statistical Manual of Mental Disorders, Fifth Edition*) (1) does not directly mention the prognosis of AD, although it does state in criterion E that 'once the stressor or its consequences have terminated, the symptoms do not persist for more than an additional 6 months'. ICD-10 (International Classification of Diseases, Tenth Revision) (2) states that the duration of symptoms does not usually exceed 6 months, except in the case of prolonged depressive reaction. Both classifications emphasize the presumptive evidence that the condition would have not arisen without the stressor.

When considering outcome, the focus in psychiatry is most commonly on symptom scores and the reduction in these with treatment. However, focusing on symptoms only is narrow and may not give a full appreciation of improvements in other domains that enrich the lives of those with mental health problems (3). For example, improvements in social functioning, including work, changes in relationships, and reduction in service utilization are among the measures worth considering. With respect to AD, usually a short-lived condition, and with a small body of research behind it, some of these have not yet been evaluated. There is an absence of measure of social functioning or relationships. Some of the variables used to evaluate outcome in AD are listed in Box 8.1.

Each of these will be discussed below.

Stability of diagnosis

Psychiatric diagnoses are notoriously unstable. This may be due to true changes; for example, depressive illness may later be replaced by

Box 8.1 Considering the course and outcome

Does the condition change into a more serious disorder, i.e., diagnostic stability?

Is the condition chronic or short-lived, i.e., morbidity?

How does the duration of hospitalization compare with that in other disorders?

How does the readmission rate in a given period compare with that in other disorders?

Is the diagnosis associated with serious comorbidity?

How labour-intensive is the management of AD compared to that in other disorders?

How does the mortality rate compare to that in other disorders?

a diagnosis of bipolar disorder when the hypomanic/manic features appear. Depressive illness may later change to alcohol dependence syndrome when the person discloses hitherto concealed alcohol misuse. The various approaches to the use of specific diagnostic criteria, as well as the clinical settings in which they are applied (e.g., inpatient versus outpatient), may also contribute to this instability. This is best exemplified by the position with AD which, once the required number of symptoms are present, and when the 2-week threshold is reached, it changes to major depression.

One group (4) conducted a study in over 10,000 subjects in different settings. For the settings combined, the prospective consistency (the proportion of individuals in a category who at the first evaluation retain the same diagnosis at their last evaluation, of the three most common diagnoses) was lowest for dysthymia (44.7%), next for bipolar disorder (49.4%), and best for schizophrenia (69.6%). Retrospective consistency (the proportion of individuals with a diagnosis assigned at the last evaluation who had received the same diagnosis at the first evaluation) was 43.7% for dysthymia, 45.9% for schizophrenia, and 38.1% for bipolar affective disorder. The proportion of patients who received the same diagnosis during at least 75% of their evaluations ranged from 9.8% for other specific personality disorders to 47.1% for schizophrenia, schizotypal, and delusional disorders. The main variable influencing diagnostic stability for the most prevalent psychiatric diagnoses was the clinical setting in which the patients were assessed. The inpatient setting showed the highest diagnostic stability, followed by the emergency and outpatient settings. AD was not considered in this.

Turning specifically to AD, it is likely to have poor consistency owing to the absence of specific criteria for the diagnosis and the overlap with other common mental disorders such as depressive illness and anxiety. For example, AD may be replaced by depressive episode/major depression if the symptom number and duration threshold for the latter are reached (see also Chapter 3, pp. 43–4, Vignette 2, for a critique of this). Alternatively, it may be diagnosed as 'mild' depression or one of the subthreshold disorders if the focus is on symptoms rather than on aetiology. Many with AD use alcohol for symptom relief, so substance misuse may replace the AD diagnosis, a pattern confirmed by Greenberg (5), who found that among those with an admission diagnosis of AD, 40% left with a different diagnosis and only 18% were given that diagnosis on readmission. Many had a comorbid diagnosis of substance misuse. The depressant effect of alcohol may initially lead to a mistaken diagnosis of AD until the alcohol use is disclosed.

The stability of various diagnoses was studied among patients admitted to hospital in the United Arab Emirates between 1993 and 1995 (6). High levels of diagnostic stability were found for schizophrenia and for bipolar and depressive disorders. A poor level of stability was found for patients with neurotic, stress-related, and adjustment disorders, ranging from zero for somatoform disorders to 50% for generalized anxiety and panic disorders, although the exact figure for AD was not provided in the study. More recently, a retrospective study of those with an admission diagnosis of AD found that when the ICD-10 criteria were applied by two independent assessors, 64% met the diagnostic criteria for that disorder (7). The authors drew attention to the clear limitations of the current diagnostic criteria and the challenges they posed to the validity and usefulness of this concept (see also Chapter 1, p. 6, for a critique of this issue). A study of case register diagnoses of more than 1,400 patients admitted more than twice found that the diagnostic stability was highest for psychotic disorders, and lowest for anxiety and AD, at 34%. The authors were unable to identify any variables associated with the level of stability apart from the diagnosis itself (28).

Reasons for instability of diagnosis are variable and might be due to several factors. These are listed in Box 8.2. The first is that many psychiatrists have limited familiarity with AD and may instead diagnose a more well-defined condition on readmission. This is one of the consequences of having poorly delineated criteria. The second reason is that once the duration or symptom threshold for another condition is reached, the diagnosis will automatically change from AD to, usually, either major depression or generalized anxiety disorder, even when the stressor is still present and AD might be a more appropriate diagnosis. So in these circumstances the diagnostic instability reflects the rigid application of the current criteria in DSM-5 and ICD-10. The third explanation is that the misuse of alcohol to deal with stressors is commonly not disclosed in the initial phase of treatment, and what appears to be an AD may be a manifestation of the depressant effects of alcohol or other substances. Since diagnoses are made at a single point in time, at least in the early stages of contact with the patient, what appears to be an AD is in fact a depressive episode/major depression/generalized anxiety disorder in evolution, which is clarified with further observation over time. Finally, what appears to be AD may in fact represent a long-standing pattern of maladaptive coping strategies that, in their totality, are best viewed as a personality disorder. This is most likely to occur when the patient is previously unknown to the psychiatrist.

Box 8.2 Reasons for diagnostic instability

Lack of knowledge of AD and vague criteria
Rigid adherence to the diagnostic criteria for threshold disorders
Undisclosed alcohol and other substance misuse
What seems to be AD is an evolving depressive episode or some other diagnosis
Personality disorder

Comorbidity

Few studies have examined the disorders that are comorbid with AD, an exercise that is hampered by the fact that the criteria for AD appear to preclude DSM Axis 1 comorbidity. ICD-10 is silent on comorbidity with AD, while DSM-5 criterion C states, 'The stress-related disturbance does not meet the criteria for another mental disorder and is not merely an exacerbation of a pre-existing mental disorder.' In the subsequent general description, it clarifies this further by stating, 'Adjustment disorders can be diagnosed in addition to another mental disorder only if the latter does not explain the particular symptoms that occur in reaction to the stressor'. The following example is offered of a person losing a job and developing AD and at the same time having a diagnosis of obsessive compulsive disorder. A further example is then given, which may appear contradictory when first read: 'An individual may have a depressive or bipolar disorder and an adjustment disorder as long as the criteria for both are met'. Presumably this refers to a person with a well-controlled pre-existing disorder, accompanied by heightened symptomatology or dysfunction in response to a discrete, stressful event such as a job loss or relationship breakdown.

Despite the paucity of studies on comorbidity, one particular study found that almost half of the patients exhibited comorbidity with major depression or PTSD (post-traumatic stress disorder) (8). Surprisingly, complicated grief and AD were not significantly comorbid. These findings should not be surprising since comorbidity is commonly associated with all psychiatric disorders and in some instances, as the authors point out, may represent the co-occurrence with another disorder of different aetiology.

What happens over time?

There have been few studies on the prognosis of those with adjustment disorder, and most of these are old.

The DSM-IV-TR (text revision) (9) criterion E for AD implies a good long-term outcome by stating that 'once the stressor (or its consequences) has terminated, the symptoms do not persist for more than an additional 6 months'. One landmark study (10) demonstrated this by showing that prognosis was favourable for adults and that at

5-year follow up, 71% were well, 21% developed either major depression or alcohol abuse, and 8% had some intervening problem. By contrast, among adolescents, many major psychiatric illnesses eventually occur as they age. In adolescents at 5-year follow up, only 44% were without a psychiatric diagnosis, 13% had an intervening psychiatric illness, and 43% had developed major psychiatric morbidity (e.g., schizophrenia, schizoaffective disorder, major depression, bipolar disorder, substance abuse, personality disorders). The predictors of major pathology at the 5-year follow up among adolescents included the presence of behavioural problems and the chronicity of the symptoms. The number and type of symptoms were less useful as predictors of future outcome. Similarly, other studies (11, 12) observed that a significant number of AD patients either do not improve or grow worse in adolescence and early adult life. However, one study (13) examined children and youth (aged 8–13 years) for up to 8 years and observed that, after controlling for the effects of comorbidity, AD did not predict later dysfunction.

A recent study (27) sheds more light on what happens to those with AD over time. The study population comprised over 800 subjects followed up post-injury. However, no diagnosis was made until 3 months post event, thus potentially excluding at least some with AD having an onset before that. A further caveat is that the measure of AD was a schedule that is usually used to evaluate PTSD symptoms. Thus, this study may not have been measuring AD as it is currently understood in ICD-10 and DSM-5. A prevalence of AD of 18.9% at 3 months was identified and almost 33% continued to have AD at 12 months, while a further 20% developed another unspecified disorder. The remainder of those diagnosed with AD (47%) had no disorder at 12 months. It showed that having a diagnosis of AD at the 3-month point, compared to no diagnosis, increased the risk of having AD at 12 months, although it is not clear whether this chronicity was due to the ongoing impact of the injuries causing pain, and physical incapacity. Having a diagnosis of AD significantly increased the risk of having any psychiatric disorder at 12 months. Also, new cases of AD developed beyond the 3-month period. These are new findings that challenge, among others, the view that AD is a short-lived condition. It needs to be replicated using criteria that match the current concept of AD as well as that proposed in ICD-11 (and used in the above study). Thus, the figure of 47% showing symptom resolution, while much lower than that described in other studies (10), must be interpreted in light of the methodology of this study.

Duration of hospitalization and readmission rates

Turning to the duration of hospitalization, some (5) have found this to be shorter in those with AD, and also that hospitalization was associated with more presenting suicidality than comparison diagnostic groups. In addition, outpatient treatment has been found to be shorter for those with AD than for those with other diagnoses (25), and this same study also revealed that 16% of patients required treatment for more than 1 year, demonstrating that AD can be a chronic condition in a minority of subjects Readmission rates also provide information on outcome. Greenberg et al.'s study (5) also revealed that adults, but not adolescents, with an admission diagnosis of AD had fewer readmissions over the following 2-year period, and this pattern was replicated when 10 years of readmission data was studied (14). Among various psychiatric diagnoses, AD had the lowest readmission rates. Initial psychological recovery from an AD may be attributable to removal of the stressor or recovery from the effects of the stressor. This may explain the findings that prisoners who developed AD after being placed in solitary confinement experienced symptom resolution shortly after their release (15). Others (7) also found that 19.8% of patients with an ICD-10 diagnosis of AD were readmitted within 5 years, and of these, 9.9% showed a change in diagnosis.

Suicidal behaviour

Suicidal behaviour is one of the behaviours associated with a diagnosis of AD (18, 19, 60). This is of great importance in terms of the distress to the patients and to their families that is associated with self-harm. There are obvious resource implications also since self-harm places an additional burden on the psychiatric services over and above that of the underlying condition itself.

Yet the quality of many of the studies examining the relationship between self-harm and AD is poor: some are retrospective, the diagnosis of AD appears to have been made using uncertain criteria, sample sizes are small, and it is possible that the diagnosis of AD is applied inappropriately to those experiencing the rapid mood shifts that are inherent to borderline personality disorder. AD should not be diagnosed in these circumstances. For example, one such retrospective case-note study found that among patients with a diagnosis of AD assessed at a university hospital, 67% had a DSM Axis 2 diagnosis of either antisocial or borderline personality disorder, 60% had a past history of suicide attempts, and high levels of substance abuse and compulsory hospital admissions were also reported (18). The suicidal group also had high levels of child sexual abuse. In a further study (19) among consecutively referred young people aged under 22 years with a diagnosis of AD, 25% had a history of self-harm. Despite the small numbers in this study, the multivariate analysis identified the suicidal group as particularly dysfunctional with high levels of prior psychiatric treatment, poorer social function than their non-suicidal counterparts, and higher levels of restlessness with suicide in others acting as a stressor when compared to their non-suicidal counterparts (19). Among those presenting to the emergency department for evaluation after an episode of self-harm (60), almost one-third were given a clinical diagnosis of AD. Following outpatient treatment, up to 14% of those with AD engaged in self-harm behaviour (25).

These studies, notwithstanding their limitations, point to the particular role of self-harm in those with AD as indicating higher levels of dysfunction compared to those with AD who do not self-harm. However, further studies using better methodology and taking care to exclude those with a diagnosis of borderline personality disorder are required if the noxious contribution of self-harm behaviour in those with a diagnosis of AD is to be confirmed with greater certainty than the present studies permit.

Despite the association between self-harm and a diagnosis of AD discussed above, the picture is muddied when other conditions such as major depression are compared to AD. One study (26) found that a lifetime history of suicide attempts was much higher in those with major depression (27%) and dysthymic disorder (17%) than in those with AD

(4%), while the figures for suicidal thoughts were 57%, 55%, and 21%, with AD having the lowest prevalence. It also appears that suicidal behaviour behaves differently in those with AD than in those with other diagnoses. It occurs at an earlier stage with AD (at 1 month) compared to depression (3 months), borderline personality disorder (30 months), and schizophrenia (47 months) (16). Casey (17) identified self-harm as occurring at a lower symptom threshold in those with AD compared to ICD-10-defined depressive episode and with lower suicide intent scores in the objective circumstances measures.

In terms of the neurochemical variables of AD patients of all ages who had attempted suicide, the biological correlates are consistent with the more major psychiatric disorders (20). Attempters exhibited lower platelet monoamine oxidase activity, higher 3-methoxy-4-hydroxyphenylglycol (MHPG) activity, and higher cortisol levels than control subjects. Although these findings differ from the lower MHPG and cortisol levels found in patients with major depression and suicidality, they are similar to the observations in other major stress-related conditions.

Contrary to the belief that AD is located at the 'mild' end of the psychiatric spectrum compared to schizophrenia, studies of AD and suicide suggest that in this measure at least it is not 'mild'. A psychological autopsy study among adolescents identified AD as the diagnosis in up to one-third of young people who die by suicide (21). In this group, suicidal thinking was brief and evolved rapidly and without warning, complicating an attempt at timely intervention (22). Among adults, AD was among the most common diagnoses in those dying by suicide in some cultures (23), with alcohol dependence syndrome and adjustment disorder being diagnosed in 16% and 15%, respectively. A study of self-immolating patients with high suicide intent admitted to a burns unit with their injuries (some of whom died as a result) found a diagnosis of AD in 67% compared to 10% in the control population from the general population (24).

Conclusion

The diagnostic stability of AD has been shown to be poor, as for most non-psychotic mental disorders. One reason for this is likely to be the absence of any specific diagnostic criteria and the change in diagnosis once the time threshold of 2 weeks is reached. The criteria for AD specify that the prognosis is good and that symptoms resolve once the stressor or its consequences is removed. This has been confirmed by follow-up studies (10) showing that, over time, those with AD remain well—apart from adolescents, who have a less favourable outcome, including the development of other disorders or suicide (11, 12, 21; see also Chapter 9). Such individuals also have fewer readmissions (5) and shorter stays. Suicidal behaviour occurs earlier in the course of the disorder and at lower thresholds than with other psychiatric disorders (16, 17). Those who exhibit suicidal behaviour in association with AD have a poorer prognosis than those who do not self-harm. The studies in this area have significant methodological problems and require replication. One recent study suggests that AD may transmute into other psychiatric disorders, but this needs to be replicated also.

References

1. **American Psychiatric Association.** Diagnostic and statistical manual of mental disorders. 5th ed. Washington, DC: American Psychiatric Association; 2013.
2. **World Health Organization.** The ICD-10 classification of mental and behavioural disorders: Clinical descriptions and diagnostic guidelines. Geneva: World Health Organization; 1992.
3. **Blais MA, Sinclair SJ, Baity MR, Worth J, Weiss AP, Ball LA,** et al. Measuring outcomes in adult outpatient psychiatry. Clin Psychol Psychother. 2012;**19**(3):203–13.
4. **Baca-Garcia E, Perez-Rodriguez MM, Basurte-Villamor I.** Diagnostic stability of psychiatric disorders in clinical practice. Br J Psychiatry. 2007;**193**(3):210–16.
5. **Greenberg WM, Rosenfeld D, Ortega E.** Adjustment disorder as an admission diagnosis. Am J Psychiatry. 1995;**152**(3):459–61.
6. **Daradkeh TK, Ei-Rufaie OEF, Younis YO, Ghubash R.** The diagnostic stability of ICD-10 psychiatric diagnoses in clinical practice. Eur Psychiatry. 1997;12;136–9.
7. **Jager M, Burger D, Becker T, Frasch K.** Diagnosis of adjustment disorder: reliability of its clinical use and long-term stability. Psychopathology. 2012;**45**(5):305–9.
8. **Maercker A, Forstmeier S, Enzler A, Krüsi G, Hörler E, Maier C,** et al. Adjustment disorders, post-traumatic stress disorder, and depressive disorders in old age: findings from a community survey. Compr Psychiatry. 2008;**49**(2):113–20.

9. **American Psychiatric Association**. Diagnostic and statistical manual of mental disorders. 3rd ed, text revision. Washington, DC: American Psychiatric Association; 1987.

10. **Andreasen NC, Hoenk PR**. The predictive value of AD: a follow-up study. Am J Psychiatry. 1982;**139**:584–90.

11. **Andreasen NC, Wasek P**. AD in adolescents and adults. Arch Gen Psychiatry. 1980;**37**:1166–70.

12. **Chess S, Thomas A**. Origins and evolution of behavior disorders: from infancy to early adult life. New York: Brunner/Mazel; 1984.

13. **Kovacs M, Gatsonis C, Pollock M, Parrone PL**. A controlled prospective study of DSM-III AD in childhood: short-term prognosis and long-term predictive validity. Arch Gen Psychiatry. 1994;**51**:535–41.

14. **Jones R, Yates WR, Williams S, Zhou M, Hardman L**. Outcome for adjustment disorder with depressed mood: comparison with other mood disorders. J Affect Disord. 1999;**55**(1):55–61.

15. **Andersen HS, Sestoft D, Lillebaek T, Gabrielsen G, Hemmingsen R, Kramp P**. A longitudinal study of prisoners on remand: psychiatric prevalence, incidence and psychopathology in solitary vs. non-solitary confinement. Acta Psychiatr Scand. 2000;**102**:19–25.

16. **Runeson BS, Beskow J, Waern M**. The suicidal process in suicides among young people. Acta Psychiatr Scand. 1996;**93**:35–42.

17. **Casey P, Jabbar F, O'Leary E, Doherty AM**. Suicidal behaviours in adjustment disorder and depressive episode. J Affect Disord. 2015;**174**:441–6.

18. **Kryzhanovskaya L, Canterbury R**. Suicidal behavior in patients with AD. Crisis. 2001;**22**:125–31.

19. **Pelkonen M, Marttunen M, Henriksson M, Lönnqvist J**. Suicidality in AD—clinical characteristics of adolescent outpatients. Eur Child Adolesc Psychiatry. 2005;**14**:174–80.

20. **Tripodianakis J, Markianos M, Sarantidis D, Leotsakou C**. Neurochemical variables in subjects with adjustment disorder after suicide attempts. Eur Psychiatry. 2000;**15**(3):190–5.

21. **Lonnqvist JK, Henriksson MM, Isometsä ET, Marttunen MJ, Heikkinen ME, Aro HM, et al**. Mental disorders and suicide prevention. Psychiatry Clin Neurosci. 1995;**49**:S111–16.

22. **Portzky G, Audenaert K, van Heeringen K**. AD and the course of the suicidal process in adolescents. J Affect Disord. 2005;**87**:265–70.

23. **Manoranjitham SD, Rajkumar AP, Thangadurai P, Prasad J, Jayakaran R, Jacob KS**. Risk factors for suicide in rural south India. Br J Psychiatry. 2010;**196**:26–30.

24. **Ahmadi A, Mohammadi R, Schwebel DC, Yeganeh N, Hassanzadeh M, Bazargan-Hejazi S**. Psychiatric disorders (Axis I and Axis II) and self-immolation: a case-control study from Iran. J Forensic Sci. 2010;**55**(2):447–50.

25. **Despland JN, Monod L, Ferrero F.** Clinical relevance of adjustment disorder in DSM-III-R and DSM-IV. Compr Psychiatry 1995;**36**:454–60.

26. **Spalletta G, Troisi A, Saracco M,** et al: Symptom profile: Axis II comorbidity and suicidal behaviour in young males with DSM-III-R depressive illnesses. J Affect Disord. 1996;**39**:141–8.

27. **O'Donnell ML, Alkemade N, Creamer M, McFarlane AC, Silove D, Bryant RA,** et al. A longitudinal study of adjustment disorder after trauma exposure. Am J Psychiatry. 2016;**173**(12):1231–8.

28. **Huguelet P, Schneider El Gueddari N, Glauser D.** Stability of DSR-III-R diagnoses: study of a case register. Psychopathology. 2001;**34**:118–22.

Chapter 9

Adjustment disorders in child and adolescent psychiatry

Aisling Mulligan

"For never was a story of more woe than this of Juliet and her Romeo."
—— *William Shakespeare, Romeo and Juliet*

Clinical description of adjustment disorder in children

The diagnostic criteria for adjustment disorder (AD) in childhood are the same as those for adults—there must be a history of a stressful event and an emotional response to that stressful event, with associated psychiatric symptoms. The young person generally has no history of psychiatric symptoms prior to the stressful event. However, as in adults, there can be an increased risk of suicide in young people who have an AD.

ICD-10 (International Classification of Diseases, Tenth Revision) classifies adjustment disorders as 'Neurotic, stress-related and somatoform disorders' (F40–F48), with many subtypes of AD listed under the heading 'Reaction to severe stress, and adjustment disorder' (F43.20–F43.28). The onset of symptoms must be within 1 month of the stressful event, but symptoms must not persist beyond 6 months of the stressor, except in cases of 'Adjustment disorder with prolonged depressive symptoms'.

ICD-10 requires that for a diagnosis of an AD there must have been the experience of an identifiable psycho-social stressor or (which may not be of a catastrophic type), within one month of the onset of symptoms as well as subjective distress or emotional disturbance. Symptoms found in any of the affective disorders, any of the neurotic, stress-related and somatoform disorders or conduct disorders may be present so long as the criteria of an individual disorder are not fulfilled. Symptoms may be variable in form and severity symptoms. The predominant features may then also be specified—for example, depressive (brief or prolonged), or mixed anxiety and depressive, with predominant disturbance of other emotions. Of note, in children, regressive behaviour such as thumb-sucking and bedwetting can occur.

Adjustment disorder in DSM-5 is categorized under Trauma and Stressor-Related Disorders. The diagnostic criteria are similar to those in ICD-10, but the timeline requirements are slightly different: there must be the development of emotional or behavioural symptoms in response to an identifiable stressor(s) occurring within 3 *months* of the onset of the stressor. It is also required that there is impairment, that the symptoms are not part of normal bereavement, and that the symptoms disappear within 6 months of the cessation of the stressor.

Young people can be particularly sensitive to stress. They are developmentally less prepared than adults for the traumas often associated with adult life, such as the trauma of a relationship break-up, bullying, exam pressures, and the challenges of a physical-illness diagnosis. Teenage life is a time of differentiating from parents, thus young people may not seek the support of parents or other adults if they are challenged. More recently, challenges associated with social media profiles and cyberbullying can be stressors for young people.

Andreasen & Hoenk (1) studied the validity of the diagnosis of AD by assessing the status, at 5-year follow up, of 100 patients given the diagnosis of AD. This study strongly supports the validity of the diagnosis among adults, but only partially among adolescents. At 5 years, just 57% of adolescents were well at follow up, compared with 79% of adults.

Pelkonen et al. (2) explored the clinical characteristics of 89 young people aged 12–22 years with DSM-III-R (*Diagnostic and Statistical Manual of Mental Disorders, revised Third Edition*) AD who were referred for outpatient psychiatric secondary care in Finland. They found that AD with depressed mood was the most common sub-class of the disorder. It was found that 50% of the young people with AD had experienced parental divorce, and that those with AD were more likely than those with other non-psychotic psychiatric disorders to be admitted to hospital. In total, 25% of the group reported sui-cidal threats, suicidal attempts, or suicidal thinking. It was noted that school-related stressors, problems with the law, and restless-ness characterized the males, while parental illness and internalizing symptoms characterized the females (2). Pelkonen et al. (2) noted that young people report stressors related to their parents, their peer group, and their school/work, and that only 6.7% of young people reported only one stressor.

It has been shown that adolescents with AD tend to have many be-havioural symptoms, while adults with AD may have many depres-sive symptoms (3). Behavioural symptoms reported by Pelkonen et al. (2) included aggressive behaviour, school absence, and alcohol misuse. However, they noted that young people with AD were less se-verely impaired than young people with other non-psychotic psychi-atric disorders.

Adjustment disorder case vignettes

Case one

A 15-year-old female (Ann) presented to A&E, accompanied by her concerned parents, with a history of a paracetamol overdose that day, and thoughts of not wanting to live. The young person had become upset, withdrawn, and disin-terested in school and friends over the previous week, after her boyfriend of 10 months ended their relationship. Her sleep was disturbed and her appetite was poor. Prior to this she had been generally well and a high performer in school and in extra-curricular activities, and had a large circle of friends. Her former boyfriend was 18 years old and had been offered a college place in another city. Her mother described him as Ann's 'first love'. Ann had no previous history of self-harm or low mood, and her current presentation was markedly different to her 'usual self'.

On mental state examination it was noted that Ann was disinterested in her physical appearance, and that her mood was low. She expressed thoughts of self-harm and recurrently expressed a wish to talk to her former boy-friend by telephone. She believed that she could not go on with life if they could not get back together. She had no hope for the future and was not interested in her usual activities. Ann was diagnosed with an AD with brief depressive reaction (F43.20 using ICD-10).

Ann was admitted to a paediatric ward for one-to-one observation, in view of the risk of self-harm or suicide. Alternative coping strategies were explored with Ann while she was in hospital, and she was taught some mindfulness skills. A safety plan was agreed between Ann and her parents—she agreed to confide in her mother if she felt unwell or suicidal. Her mood gradually improved while in hospital, and after 2 days she was fit for discharge. Close supervision by her parents was recommended on discharge from hospital, as well as activity planning as a distraction technique. She was advised not to take alcohol or drugs in view of the possibility of this precipitating an episode of low mood. A follow-up appointment at her local Child and Adolescent Mental Health Service (CAMHS) was organized for one week after discharge—at that appointment it was noted that Ann was back at school, and an improvement in her mood was noted. She was no longer suicidal. After one further follow-up appointment, Ann was discharged from CAMHS.

Case two

Tom is a 13-year-old male who was brought to a CAMHS clinic for assessment following an episode where he was found walking on a viaduct, contemplating jumping from the bridge, which would have undoubtedly resulted in death. This event occurred 3 weeks after he was taken into the care of the state, and was brought to live in a care home with other teenagers, having lived with his mother up to that date. Both his parents were drug addicts and Tom had been fending for himself while living with his mother, not attending school, and stealing food to survive. A concerned neighbour had contacted community care services, who had organized his transfer to the care home.

Immediately prior to walking on the viaduct, Tom had made a phone call to his father, and expressed a desire to live with his father instead of with his mother or in the care home. However, his father pointed out that this was not possible.

At interview, Tom was dismissive of symptoms of distress or low mood and was critical of the move to the care home and the staff there. He denied all symptoms of depression. The care home staff noted, however, that he had a history of diffi-cult behaviour patterns while in the care home, not following instructions from staff, not attending school, and spending prolonged periods of time on the street. The care staff were concerned that he may have been at risk of getting involved in criminal activity.

Tom was diagnosed with an AD with predominant disturbance of con-duct (F43.24 using ICD-10). He was offered the opportunity to attend some individual therapy sessions to allow him to discuss the recent changes in his life, and he was offered the opportunity to join a young person's skills-based training programme, which was part of the dialectical behaviour programme in the CAMHS clinic. However, Tom did not want to attend any services at CAMHS. Staff in the care home were informed of his diagnosis and were given clear instructions to supervise him closely, as he was considered to remain at high risk of attempted suicide. A busy schedule of activity, including school and after-school activities, was recommended for Tom, especially in view of the risk of him developing a conduct disorder. He was advised not to take alcohol or drugs in view of the possibility of this leading to an episode of low mood, with associated self-harm.

Tom subsequently returned to school and was noted to have developed a confiding relationship with one of the teachers. He had no further episodes of deliberate self-harm.

Prevalence of adjustment disorder in children

A review of the literature regarding adjustment disorders in children and adolescents concluded that the condition is common and has significant morbidity, with a poor outcome in children and adolescents (4). It appears from epidemiological studies that the prevalence rates of adjustment disorders are lower in young people than in older adults. While the overall prevalence of AD may be relatively low, it should be noted that young people with AD frequently present to psychiatric services, with rates of 12– 31% of those presenting to psychiatric services having a diagnosis of AD (see Table 9.1).

An epidemiological study looking at psychiatric diagnoses in a sample from a birth cohort of 60,000 children aged 8–9 years in Finland found that 3.4% of children had a diagnosis of 'adjustment disorder with mixed disturbance of emotion and conduct,' the third most common clinical disorder in this age-group, after attention deficit hyperactivity disorder (ADHD) (7%) and dysthymia (4.6%) (5). However, a recent epidemiological study from Germany on the prevalence of AD found a lower prevalence rate of 0.2% in young people aged 14–29 years, with the rates in young people lower than the rates of AD in those aged 30–59 years (1.7%) or those aged 60–95 years (1.3%) (6). Similarly, an increase in the incidence of AD as people got older was noted in a Danish registry study of patients diagnosed

Table 9.1 Prevalence and incidence studies on adjustment disorders in children

Author	Location	Prevalence rate	Comment
Almqvist et al. (5)	Finland	3.4%	8–9 year olds
Maercker et al. (6)	Germany	0.2%	14–29 years
		Incidence rate	
Pelkonen et al. (2)	Finland	31%	Prospective A&E study, 12–22 year olds
Lee et al. (9)	Canada	29%	Prospective study, presenting to emergency Child and Adolescent Psychiatry setting
Grudnikoff et al. (11)	USA	24%	Psychiatric paediatric emergency dept
Aebi et al. (12)	Switzerland	12%	Child psychiatry public clinic, 5–18 year olds
Di Lorenzo et al. (13)	Italy	29.3% of females 7.6% of males	Retrospective study of 14–18 year olds admitted to adolescent inpatient psychiatric service
Kovacs et al. (14)	USA	33%	Children newly diagnosed with diabetes Type 1
Piyavhatkul et al. (15)	Southern Thailand	9.6%	Child survivors of the Asian tsunami

with ICD-10 adjustment disorders or with stress reactions between 1995 and 2011 (7). It was found that the rates of these diagnoses increased throughout teenage life into the early thirties, and that the rates were considerably higher in females than in males (60% vs 40%) (7).

While the prevalence of adjustment disorders in children is relatively low, the incidence is higher, reflecting that many young people recover completely from their symptoms (8). A considerable number of young people presenting to A&E and to psychiatric services fulfil a diagnosis of AD.

A prospective study of 12–22 year olds presenting consecutively to psychiatric outpatients in Finland found that AD was the second most common non-psychotic presentation, affecting 31% of 290 consecutively referred patients (2). In this study, Pelkonen et al. further examined the characteristics of the 89 patients with AD and noted that compared to other non-psychotic patients, those with AD were predominantly female and had less severe psychosocial impairment (2). A Canadian prospective study of 170 patients (mean age 12 years) referred from a paediatric emergency setting to a child and adolescent psychiatry service found that AD was the most common diagnosis, at a rate of 29% (9).

A study of 241 consults in 1 year to a child and adolescent psychiatry service in a paediatric university hospital found that the most frequent reason for consultation was mood complaints, with major depressive disorder and AD the most frequent preliminary diagnosis (10). Many consultations related to mood symptoms in conjunction with a neurological, malignancy, or endocrine diagnosis. Similarly, 24% of young people presenting to a US psychiatric paediatric emergency department (11) had a diagnosis of AD.

It was noted that 43 of 354 children (12%) aged 5–18 years (mean age 10.5 years) referred to a child psychiatry public clinic in Switzerland had a diagnosis of AD assigned by a clinician (12). However, this may not reflect the true rate of AD in children presenting to the clinic—a large number of children were excluded from this study due to incomplete information or lack of parental interest in the study. A retrospective study of the diagnosis and characteristics of adolescents aged 14–18 years admitted to an inpatient adolescent psychiatric service in Italy found that the rate of AD in females (29.3%) exceeded that in males (7.6%) (13).

AD can occur following an important diagnosis of physical illness. One study found that one-third of 92 children newly diagnosed with insulin-dependent diabetes mellitus developed an AD, with a 100% recovery rate, though in this study the diagnosis of AD was allowed up to 6 months after the diagnosis of diabetes (14).

Piyavhatkul et al. (15) studied the effects of the Asian tsunami on a group of young people who survived the tsunami in southern Thailand and found that 9.6% of the group of 94 children had a diagnosis of AD,

33% had a diagnosis of post-traumatic stress disorder, and 9.6% had a diagnosis of major depression (15).

While a research diagnosis of an AD has been shown to be relatively common in children and young people presenting for psychiatric care (2, 4, 12), the disorder may go under-reported. There is some debate about the use of the term 'adjustment disorder' in children. Similarly, in adults there can be some hesitancy with the use of this term, and one Spanish study (16) revealed that a diagnosis of AD was made by the general practitioner in just two out of 110 individuals attending their general practice. The Development and Well-Being Assessment (DAWBA) tool does not diagnose adjustment disorders (12), which may limit research on the topic in child and adolescent psychiatry in the future.

Suicide and adjustment disorder

Shakespeare's Romeo and Juliet, lovers who each died by suicide in the belief that the other had died, remind us of the acute risk of suicide in young people who have experienced an acute stressor such as relationship break-up or loss.

Pelkonen et al. (17) noted that 25% of their prospectively identified cohort of 89 patients aged 12–22 years with AD showed suicide attempts, suicidal threats, or ideation (17). They compared suicidal patients with AD with non-suicidal patients with AD and found that suicidal AD patients were characterized by previous psychiatric treatment (odds ratio (OR) = 6.1), poor psychosocial functioning at treatment entry (OR = 16.2), suicide as a stressor (OR = 33.3), dysphoric mood (OR = 6.9), and psychomotor restlessness (OR = 3.7) (17). Portzky et al. (18) interviewed relatives of 19 adolescents who completed suicide and found that those with a history of AD had a shorter period of suicidal behaviour prior to suicide and fewer symptoms of behavioural or emotional difficulties in early adolescence than those who completed suicide with a prior history of depression or other psychiatric disorders.

A comparison study of 97 adolescents with AD attending a Spanish public mental health service with a similar number of adolescents without AD found that girls with AD reported significantly higher symptoms of suicidal ideation and suicidal intent than (a) boys with AD and (b) girls without AD (19). In contrast to this, no differences were found in the community between boys with AD and boys without AD in terms of their scores on suicidal ideation or intent. In the sample of adolescents with AD, suicidal symptoms were reported by 27% of girls and 18% of boys, although only 6% of the girls and none of the boys presented clear suicidal tendencies (19).

The presence of AD was significantly associated with suicidal ideation in a retrospective study of children aged up to 18 years who presented to a US paediatric emergency room (11). A total of 1,062 young people were assessed, of whom 25% had suicidal ideation/thinking or had suicidal behaviour. Moreover, 254 young people were diagnosed with an AD, which was significantly associated with suicidal ideation. The authors of this study recommended that those with adjustment disorders should be closely monitored owing to suicidal risk.

We can conclude that young people with AD are at risk of suicide—with 25% of them reporting suicidal thoughts or acts—and that they may have a brief disturbance of behaviour and mental state prior to suicide, and that girls in particular with AD may report suicidal symptoms.

Prognosis of adjustment disorder in childhood

While most adolescents recover from AD (20, 21), there is an association with the onset of other psychiatric illnesses, including major depressive disorder, behavioural disorders, psychotic disorders, and personality disorders. There is considerable morbidity associated with a diagnosis of AD in adolescence (4), while a diagnosis of AD in childhood is associated with repeat utilization of child psychiatry emergency services (22). In the short term, adolescents with AD have an increased risk of suicide and of suicidal behaviour, as described above.

The 5-year follow-up study of 100 patients with AD, by Andreasen & Hoenk (1), found that the prognosis for adolescents is not as good as that for adults. Both the rate of psychiatric disorders at 5-year follow up and the nature of the disorders differed in adolescents in comparison to adults. Just 57% of adolescents were well at follow up compared to 79% of adults at 5 years. Adults who were ill developed either major depression or alcoholism, whereas adolescents developed schizo-phrenia, schizoaffective disorder, major depression, bipolar disorder, antisocial personality disorder, alcoholism, and drug use disorder. For adolescents, the presence of behavioural symptoms predicted a poor outcome (1).

Kovacs et al. (8) compared 30 children aged 8–13 years with a diagnosis of DSM-III AD with three clinically significant symptoms with a similar group of children who had other psychiatric disorders, and followed up both groups for 7–8 years, on average. They found that 97% of patients with AD recovered (from AD), and that the disorder had a median episode duration of 7 months. They also found that patients with AD and the control group had similar rates of new psychiatric disorders and other dysfunctional outcomes over the follow-up period, in contrast to the findings of Andreasen & Hoenk (1). Kovacs et al. (8) concluded that, controlling for the effects of comorbidity, AD in young patients does not predict later dysfunction.

In a follow-up study comparing young adults who had a history of major depressive disorder in adolescence with young adults who had a history of AD in adolescence, it has been shown that those who presented with AD were at increased risk of major depressive dis-order as young adults, with the risk of developing major depressive disorder similar to the risk in those who experienced major depressive disorder in adolescence (23).

Kovacs et al. (20) performed a prospective, longitudinal study to explore the characteristics and diagnostic validity of 'major de-pressive disorder', 'dysthymic disorder', and 'adjustment disorder with depressed mood' in a school-aged cohort. They found that the three disorders differed in terms of age at onset and pattern of re-covery. They found that the prognosis for AD was good, with 90% of children achieving remission from symptoms within 9 months.

They also found that the three disorders had different levels of risk in terms of developing a subsequent major depressive disorder, with 'adjustment disorder with depressed mood' associated with a lower risk of developing a major depressive disorder than the risk for young people who had already experienced a major depressive disorder (24). It was also noted that children with 'adjustment disorder with depressed mood' had less comorbid anxiety than children with depressive disorder or dysthymia (25). Children with 'adjustment disorder and depressed mood' also had less subsequent suicidal behaviour than children who had major depressive disorder or children who had dysthymia (26). These studies indicated the validity of the diagnostic category of 'adjustment disorder and depressed mood' and serve to inform us about the prognosis of the disorder. Kovacs et al. (14) suggest that the prognosis for AD may be related to the stress which has precipitated the disorder.

A follow-up study of DSM-III diagnoses of 19 children with AD who had presented to a community speech and language clinic found that none of the children continued to have AD upon follow up 4 years later (21). However, 11 children had a diagnosis of DSM-III Attention Deficit Disorder with Hyperactivity at follow up, two had oppositional disorder, and six had overanxious disorder. It appeared that children recovered from the AD but that they were highly inclined to have developed a behavioural disorder.

A Danish registry follow-up study of 485 children who had been admitted to inpatient psychiatric care over a 3-year period, and followed up approximately 16 years later, found that girls with AD had higher risks of admission to psychiatric hospital in young adulthood (aged 16+ years) with a diagnosis of personality disorders and psychosis (27).

We can conclude that a diagnosis of AD in adolescence is often associated with a resolution of symptoms of AD, but that the young person is at increased risk of other psychiatric conditions later in life. The prognosis for adolescents with AD is considered to be worse than that for adults with AD in view of this increased risk of other psychiatric disorders. The diagnosis of AD predicts the need for more psychiatric services in the future.

Factors predisposing to the development of adjustment disorder

A limited number of studies have been conducted on possible factors predisposing to the development of AD. Varma et al. (28) studied levels of glycoproteins and glycosaminoglycans in children with schizophrenia, conduct disorder, and AD, and in those with no disorder. The findings revealed a raised galactosamine level in children with AD compared to those with no disorder, and it has been hypothesized that this may be related to stress in the environment (28). Children with schizophrenia and with conduct disorder also had biochemical abnormalities (28).

Lung et al. (29) examined the association between the style of parental bonding and personality characteristics, and AD—with and without hyperventilation syndrome—in a study of 917 males, 156 with AD. They proposed that 'parental bonding affected personality characteristics, personality characteristics affected mental health condition, and mental health condition affected the development of hyperventilation or adjustment disorder'. Males with AD without hyperventilation perceived less paternal care; males with AD with hyperventilation perceived more maternal protection than those with AD and those in the control group (29). Simmen-Janevska et al. (30) reviewed the literature on the relationship between motivational skills and response to traumatic stress, and also the influence of traumatic stress on the ability to motivate oneself. They concluded that 'motivational constructs seem to predict posttraumatic stress over the life span'.

The concept of resilience is important in child and adolescent psychiatry—we do not yet fully understand why some young people respond to stress by developing an AD or other mental health condition while others respond by adapting to the stressor. This is an area that warrants further research.

Management of adjustment disorders in children

There is limited formal research into treatments for AD in young people. However, there is a considerable body of research regarding the management of deliberate self-harm and of suicidal thinking, which may occur in association with an AD (31).

As with many presenting conditions in child and adolescent psychiatry, a risk assessment followed by psycho-education of the patient and carers about the young person's condition is important. All children and young people presenting with an AD should be assessed for suicidal ideation and managed appropriately. Some young people with suicidal tendencies are admitted to hospital overnight or for a brief admission for 'crisis intervention', often being admitted to paediatric hospitals under intensive observation (one-to-one special observation) rather than being admitted to an adolescent psychiatric inpatient bed.

Brief psychodynamic therapy and other psychotherapeutic interventions have been used to treat AD in adults (32). There is little or no research available on the use of specific therapies in children with AD. However, as young people with adjustment disorders present frequently to psychiatry services either via emergency room presentations or via child psychiatry outpatient services with symptoms of low mood or suicidal thinking, many of these young people receive follow-up therapeutic or mood monitoring services at mental health services. A recent analysis of the services offered to adolescents presenting with depressive symptoms noted that those with a diagnosis of AD were often offered therapy/services (33).

A recent publication describes an internet-based intervention developed for adults with AD which provides skills that have much in common with the theories of cognitive–behavioural therapy, mindfulness, and relaxation techniques (34). A randomized controlled trial of this intervention is planned, but the results are not yet available (34). If this is an effective intervention in adults it may also be effective in children and adolescents with AD—and its delivery via the internet may be more popular with young people than a face-to-face therapeutic service. As the use of social media and the internet is so important to young people, it is important to consider the possibility of delivering therapeutic services to young people with an AD via such avenues, for example via an app on a mobile device. An association between the use of social media and suicidal thinking has been revealed in a large study of adolescents in Canada (35). It is possible that, by providing services via the internet or social media, those services will actually target those adolescents who are most in need of therapeutic services.

Treatment as usual offered for low mood or suicidal ideation in child and adolescent mental health services may include practical measures such as removing or reducing the effect of the stressor—for example, by requesting that an adult intervene if the young person is a victim of bullying or cyberbullying. Education of adults on the safe use and monitoring of social media may be beneficial. The skills taught in dialectical behaviour therapy may be useful to the adolescent with thoughts of self-harm and AD. Parent training on the management of self-harm may also be provided, or parents may be referred to a parent support group. Medication use is generally not indicated for the treatment of AD in children. However, as many young people who present with an AD later develop a depressive episode, they may need mood monitoring with the possibility of later being treated with cognitive–behavioural therapy or a selective serotonin reuptake inhibitor for a depressive episode.

Conclusions

Adjustment disorders in young people are a relatively common reason for presentation to emergency psychiatric services. The risks of developing an AD increase as young people get older. The diagnostic criteria for an AD in young people are the same as for adults, though the profile of underlying stressors varies. The diagnosis is usually self-limiting. However, there is a risk of suicide and of suicidal behaviour and ideation, which must be carefully managed. For those young people who recover from the AD, it appears that they retain an increased risk of other psychiatric disorders, and that this risk of comorbid conditions exceeds the risk of comorbid conditions in adults. Hence, the presence of an AD in adolescence is associated with more psychiatric presentations in later life.

References

1. **Andreasen NC, Hoenk PR.** The predictive value of adjustment disorders: a follow-up study. Am J Psychiatry. 1982;**139**(5):584–90.
2. **Pelkonen M, Marttunen M, Henriksson M, Lonnqvist J.** Adolescent adjustment disorder: precipitant stressors and distress symptoms of 89 outpatients. Eur Psychiatry. 2007;**22**(5):288–95.

3. **Andreasen NC, Wasek P.** Adjustment disorders in adolescents and adults. Arch Gen Psychiatry. 1980;**37**(10):1166–70.

4. **Newcorn JH, Strain J.** Adjustment disorder in children and adolescents. J Am Acad Child Adolesc Psychiatry. 1992;**31**(2):318–26.

5. **Almqvist F, Puura K, Kumpulainen K, Tuompo-Johansson E, Henttonen I, Huikko E,** et al. Psychiatric disorders in 8-9-year-old children based on a diagnostic interview with the parents. Eur Child Adolesc Psychiatry. 1999;**8**(suppl 4):17–28.

6. **Maercker A, Forstmeier S, Pielmaier L, Spangenberg L, Brahler E, Glaesmer H.** Adjustment disorders: prevalence in a representative nationwide survey in Germany. Soc Psychiatry Psychiatr Epidemiol. 2012;**47**(11):1745–52.

7. **Gradus JL, Bozi I, Antonsen S, Svensson E, Lash TL, Resick PA,** et al. Severe stress and adjustment disorder diagnoses in the population of Denmark. J Trauma Stress. 2014;**27**(3):370–4.

8. **Kovacs M, Gatsonis C, Pollock M, Parrone PL.** A controlled prospective study of DSM-III adjustment disorder in childhood. Short-term prognosis and long-term predictive validity. Arch Gen Psychiatry. 1994;**51**(7):535–41.

9. **Lee J, Korczak D.** Emergency physician referrals to the pediatric crisis clinic: reasons for referral, diagnosis and disposition. J Can Acad Child Adolesc Psychiatry. 2010;**19**(4):297–302.

10. **Ríos Pelati M, Estremera Mdel M, Martinez K, Pagán A.** Epidemiological profile of psychiatry consultations at the University Pediatric Hospital. Bol Asoc Med P R. 2009;**101**(1):13–17.

11. **Grudnikoff E, Soto EC, Frederickson A, Birnbaum ML, Saito E, Dicker R,** et al. Suicidality and hospitalization as cause and outcome of pediatric psychiatric emergency room visits. Eur Child Adolesc Psychiatry. 2015;**24**(7):797–814.

12. **Aebi M, Kuhn C, Metzke CW, Stringaris A, Goodman R, Steinhausen HC.** The use of the development and well-being assessment (DAWBA) in clinical practice: a randomized trial. Eur Child Adolesc Psychiatry. 2012;**21**(10):559–67.

13. **Di Lorenzo R, Cimino N, Di Pietro E, Pollutri G, Neviani V, Ferri P.** A 5-year retrospective study of demographic, anamnestic, and clinical factors related to psychiatric hospitalizations of adolescent patients. Neuropsychiatr Dis Treat. 2016;**12**:191–201.

14. **Kovacs M, Ho V, Pollock MH.** Criterion and predictive validity of the diagnosis of adjustment disorder: a prospective study of youths with new-onset insulin-dependent diabetes mellitus. Am J Psychiatry. 1995;**152**(4):523–8.

15. **Piyavhatkul N, Pairojkul S, Suphakunpinyo C.** Psychiatric disorders in tsunami-affected children in Ranong province, Thailand. Med Princ Pract. 2008;**17**(4):290–5.

16. **Fernandez A, Mendive JM, Salvador-Carulla L, Rubio-Valera M, Luciano JV, Pinto-Meza A,** et al. Adjustment disorders in primary care: prevalence, recognition and use of services. Br J Psychiatry. 2012;**201**:137–42.

17. Pelkonen M, Marttunen M, Henriksson M, Lonnqvist J. Suicidality in adjustment disorder—clinical characteristics of adolescent outpatients. Eur Child Adolesc Psychiatry. 2005;14(3):174–80.

18. Portzky G, Audenaert K, van Heeringen K. Adjustment disorder and the course of the suicidal process in adolescents. J Affect Disord. 2005;87(2–3):265–70.

19. Ferrer L, Kirchner T. Suicidal tendency in a sample of adolescent outpatients with adjustment disorder: gender differences. Compr Psychiatry. 2014;55(6):1342–9.

20. Kovacs M, Feinberg TL, Crouse-Novak MA, Paulauskas SL, Finkelstein R. Depressive disorders in childhood. I. A longitudinal prospective study of characteristics and recovery. Arch Gen Psychiatry. 1984;41(3):229–37.

21. Cantwell DP, Baker L. Stability and natural history of DSM-III childhood diagnoses. J Am Acad Child Adolesc Psychiatry. 1989;28(5):691–700.

22. Cole W, Turgay A, Mouldey G. Repeated use of psychiatric emergency services by children. Can J Psychiatry. 1991;36(10):739–42.

23. Lewinsohn PM, Rohde P, Klein DN, Seeley JR. Natural course of adolescent major depressive disorder: I. Continuity into young adulthood. J Am Acad Child Adolesc Psychiatry. 1999;38(1):56–63.

24. Kovacs M, Feinberg TL, Crouse-Novak M, Paulauskas SL, Pollock M, Finkelstein R. Depressive disorders in childhood. II. A longitudinal study of the risk for a subsequent major depression. Arch Gen Psychiatry. 1984;41(7):643–9.

25. Kovacs M, Gatsonis C, Paulauskas SL, Richards C. Depressive disorders in childhood. IV. A longitudinal study of comorbidity with and risk for anxiety disorders. Arch Gen Psychiatry. 1989;46(9):776–82.

26. Kovacs M, Goldston D, Gatsonis C. Suicidal behaviors and childhood-onset depressive disorders: a longitudinal investigation. J Am Acad Child Adolesc Psychiatry. 1993;32(1):8–20.

27. Thomsen PH. The prognosis in early adulthood of child psychiatric patients: a case register study in Denmark. Acta Psychiatr Scand. 1990;81(1):89–93.

28. Varma R, Michos GA, Gordon BJ, Varma RS, Shirey RE. Serum glycoconjugates in children with schizophrenia and conduct and adjustment disorders. Biochem Med. 1983;30(2):206–14.

29. Lung FW, Lee TH, Huang MF. Parental bonding in males with adjustment disorder and hyperventilation syndrome. BMC Psychiatry. 2012;12:56.

30. Simmen-Janevska K, Brandstatter V, Maercker A. The overlooked relationship between motivational abilities and posttraumatic stress: a review. Eur J Psychotraumatol. 2012;3.

31. NICE (National Institute for Health and Care Excellence). Self-harm: NICE quality standard QS34. https://www.nice.org.uk/guidance/qs34

32. **Kramer U, Pascual-Leone A, Despland JN, de Roten Y.** One minute of grief: emotional processing in short-term dynamic psychotherapy for adjustment disorder. J Consult Clin Psychol. 2015;**83**(1):187–98.

33. **O'Connor BC, Lewandowski RE, Rodriguez S, Tinoco A, Gardner W, Hoagwood K,** et al. Usual care for adolescent depression from symptom identification through treatment initiation. JAMA Pediatr. 2016;**170**(4):373–80.

34. **Skruibis P, Eimontas J, Dovydaitiene M, Mazulyte E, Zelviene P, Kazlauskas E.** Internet-based modular program BADI for adjustment disorder: protocol of a randomized controlled trial. BMC Psychiatry. 2016;**16**:264.

35. **Sampasa-Kanyinga H, Hamilton HA.** Social networking sites and mental health problems in adolescents: the mediating role of cyberbullying victimization. Eur Psychiatry. 2015;**30**(8):1021–7.

Chapter 10

Adjustment disorder in disorders of intellectual development

Elspeth Bradley, Sheila Hollins, Marika Korossy, and Andrew Levitas

Introduction

Adjustment Disorder (AD) involves the development of clinically significant emotional or behavioural symptoms in response to an identifiable stressor or traumatic experience. This definition incorporates an extremely valuable diagnostic concept, suggesting that psycho-social, environmental, or health stressors, so common in the lives of people with disorders of intellectual development (DID), might be a correctable source of mental distress and psychopathology which could otherwise be mistaken for more serious mental health disorders.

Recognizing the diagnostic challenges generally in identifying psychiatric disorders in people with DID, adaptations of ICD-10 (1) criteria were published in 2001 (DC-LD) (2), and adaptations of DSM-IV-TR (3) criteria (DM-ID) (4) in 2007. DC-LD adaptations focus on the need for a multiaxial approach to understanding and diagnosing mental distress (including AD) in DID, and provide a diagnostic framework along three clinical axes (severity of DID, causes of DID, psychiatric disorders and problem behaviours) supported by crucial information (related to DID syndromes and biopsychosocial influences on health) in three appendices (see Table 10.1). Levitas & Hurley proposed adaptation of DSM-IV-TR

Table 10.1 Comparison of AD diagnostic criteria between ICD-10 & DSM-5 and adaptations of ICD & DSM for people with disorders of intellectual development (DID)

ICD-10 (1) (including Diagnostic Criteria for Research criteria)	DC-LD (2) (adaptation of ICD-10)	DM-ID (4) (adaptation of DSM-IV-TR) (3)	DSM-5 (6)
Code: F43.2	Code: IIIB5.10	Adaptations are provided for individuals with mild-to-moderate ID (MMDID); those with severe-to-profound DID (SPDID) are considered separately.	Code: 309.XX (identified by symptom manifestation 309—see below)
ONSET OF SYMPTOMS IN RESPONSE TO STRESSOR			
A: Onset of symptoms within 1 month of stressor	A: Exposure to an identified psycho-social stressor is followed within a month by onset of symptoms	A: Same as in DSM-IV-TR	A: Onset of emotional or behavioural symptoms within 3 months of stressor
Identifiable psycho-social stressor not of an unusual or catastrophic kind		As in DSM-IV-TR. Additionally, stressors may include any need for an increase in independent functioning, e.g. moves	Identifiable stressor(s)

SYMPTOMS AND IMPACT ON FUNCTIONING

B: The individual manifests symptoms or behaviour disturbance of the types found in any affective disorders (except for delusions and hallucinations), F4 disorders (neurotic, stress related, and somatoform), and conduct disorders. Predominant feature of symptoms coded as follows: F43.20: brief depressive reaction F43.21: prolonged depressive reaction F43.22—mixed anxiety & depression reaction F43.23—with predominant disturbance of other emotions F43.24—with predominant disturbance of conduct F43.25—with mixed disturbance of emotions & conduct F43.28: with other specified predominant symptoms Manifestations may include depressed mood, anxiety, worry, and feeling unable to cope, as well as some degree of disability in the performance of daily routines and interference with social functioning and performance	C: Symptoms/signs must not be a direct consequence of other psychiatric disorders, drugs, or physical disorders such as hypothyroidism D: Symptoms/signs must represent a change from the individual's pre-morbid state	B: Similar manifestation (as in DSM-IV-TR) of anxiety and depression as well as such behaviours as clinging, apparent loss of skills, withdrawal, or irritability 1: distress in excess of individuals' known baseline distress responses 2: impairment compared to individual's known baseline functioning Adaptations (for MMDID and SPDID) provided for the six subtypes of DSM-IV-TR adjustment disorder and examples given of behaviours. For example, disturbance of conduct in ID may include self-injury, threats, aggression, and property destruction (and in PSID, changes in existing patterns of any or all of these may occur). Conduct disturbance may also be observed as an increase in the frequency or severity of pre-existing maladaptive behavioural repertoires C: Adaptation: a clear history of a stressor and the differences from previous patterns seen in pre-existing Axis I & Axis II disorders must be noted Note: pre-existing disorders may not have been previously assessed E: Symptoms occur such as those found in any affective or anxiety disorders (except delusions and hallucinations), but the criteria for an individual disorder are not fulfilled	B: Clinically significant symptoms as evidenced by one or both of: 1: Marked distress in excess of what might be expected (considering context and culture) from exposure to the stressor 2: significant impairment in social, occupational, or other important areas of functioning Symptom manifestations (specifiers) are coded separately, thus: 309.0—with depressed mood 309.24—with anxiety 309.28—with mixed anxiety & depressed mood 309.3—with disturbance of conduct 309.4—with mixed disturbance of emotions and conduct 309.9—Unspecified—for maladaptive reactions not classifiable from the above C: the stress-related disturbance does not meet the criteria for another mental disorder and is not merely an exacerbation of a pre-existing mental disorder

(continued)

Table 10.1 (Continued)

ICD-10 (1) (including Diagnostic Criteria for Research criteria)	DC-LD (2) (adaptation of ICD-10)	DM-ID (4) (adaptation of DSM-IV-TR) (3)	DSM-5 (6)
DURATION OF SYMPTOMS			
C: Symptoms do not persist for longer than 6 months (except for F43.21—Prolonged depressive reaction which should not exceed 2 yrs), after cessation of the stressor or its consequences	B: Symptoms must not continue for more than 6 months after cessation of the stressor	E: Adaptation: symptoms may persist for a prolonged period in response to a chronic stressor, e.g. unrelieved inappropriate residential, educational, vocational placements; repeated care provider turnover; unrelieved peer problem exposure; or other experiences beyond the capacity of the individual to resolve independently Specifier: the assessor should determine whether the disturbance has persisted for <6 months or ≥6 months	E: Symptoms do not persist for more than 6 months after the stressor or its consequences have terminated

BEREAVEMENT

Normal bereavement reactions should not be included But grief reactions of any duration considered to be abnormal because of form or content are included and coded by one of the following F codes: F43.22; F43.23; F43.24; F43.25	No noted change from ICD-10	Adaptation: In many with ID, bereavement may take the form of anger and irritability with resulting disturbance of conduct. In these situations AD with disturbance of conduct or mixed disturbance of emotion and conduct should be diagnosed as the phenomena of normal bereavement may be significantly surpassed. Bereavement may occur in response to loss not only by death, but also by promotion, retirement, or the transfer of important caregivers (SPDID). Loss of housemates, friends, favoured staff, and even routines may be causes of grief (MMDID and SPDID)	D: Symptoms do not represent normal bereavement

STRESSORS

An appendix lists conditions that are often found in association with mental health disorders, e.g. Z codes	Appendices 1, 2, and 3 (mentioned below) provide information on circumstances that may be, or contribute to, potential stressors	Adaptation of DSM-IV-TR DSM-5 criteria provides helpful information on behaviours that might manifest in people with DID (MMDID and SPDID)	In previous DSM iterations, stressors considered relevant to the psychiatric diagnosis and subsequent treatment were listed in Axis IV. In DSM-5 the axis system has been eliminated. Psychosocial stressors are still listed using V codes; however only a few of the DSM-5 V codes are pertinent to the lives and situations of people with DID.

(continued)

Table 10.1 (Continued)

ICD-10 (1) (including Diagnostic Criteria for Research criteria)	DC-LD (2) (adaptation of ICD-10)	DM-ID (4) (adaptation of DSM-IV-TR) (3)	DSM-5 (6)
Note: (1) In children, regressive phenomena such as a return of bedwetting, babyish speech, or thumb-sucking are frequently part of the symptom pattern (2) There is no specific comment in ICD-10 about not meeting the criteria for another mental disorder	**Note:** Multiaxial classification comprises the following: Axis I: severity of LD Axis II: causes of LD Axis III: comprises the following five levels: ◆ Level A: developmental disorders ◆ Level B: psychiatric illness ◆ Level C: personality disorders ◆ Level D: problem behaviours ◆ Level E: other disorders Appendix 1: LD syndromes & behavioural phenotypes Appendix 2: other associated medical conditions Appendix 3: factors influencing health status & contact with health services		**Note:** (1) AD DSM-5 is included in the section on Trauma and Stressor-Related Disorders (was freestanding in DSM-IV-TR) (2) Other than no acute or chronic specifier, the criteria are the same as those in DSM-IV-TR

Note: People with DID not infrequently have one or several co existing psychiatric disorders. Where there is a known precipitant and the restricted time courses of onset and duration are met, AD can also occur alongside other DSM-5 disorders. Stressors in the lives of people with IDD are often unrecognised and chronic; neither ICD-10 nor DSM-5 adequately recognise these diagnostic complexities

Source: data from ICD-10: The ICD-10 Classification of Mental and Behavioural Disorders: Clinical Descriptions and Diagnostic Guidelines, Copyright (1992), WHO Organization; DC-LD: Diagnostic Criteria for Psychiatric Disorders for Use with Adults with Learning Disabilities/Mental Retardation, Copyright (2001), Royal College of Psychiatrists; Fletcher R, Loschen E, Stavrakaki C, First M [Eds], DM-ID: Diagnostic manual—intellectual disability: a textbook of diagnosis of mental disorders in persons with intellectual disability, Copyright (2007), NADD Press; Diagnostic and Statistical Manual of Mental Disorders, Fourth Edition, DSM-IV, Copyright (1994), American Psychiatric Association; Diagnostic and Statistical Manual of Mental Disorders, Fifth Edition, DSM-5, Copyright (2013), American Psychiatric Association

criteria for AD in DM-ID separately for individuals with mild-to-moderate DID (MMDID) and for those with severe-to-profound DID (SPDID; see Table 10.1) (5).

Concepts of stressors, individual responses to these stressors, and coping mechanisms are at the core of an AD diagnosis for both ICD (International Classification of Diseases) and DSM (*Diagnostic and Statistical Manual of Mental Disorders*) classificatory systems. For accurate diagnosis of AD in this population, stressors, responses, and coping mechanisms need to be considered in the context of their daily lives, personal histories, atypical development, adaptive and communication skills, and the extent to which communities in which they live, work, and play provide supportive, enabling environments (7, 8). DC-LD and DM-ID adaptations speak to these unique circumstances.

The lives of people with DID

People with DID have been marginalized and disadvantaged throughout history in many cultures (9). Negative attitudes continue to give rise to prejudice, rejection, abuse, and even hate crimes (10, 11). Socio-political influences that prioritize and underpin the development and delivery of services are similarly shaped by such attitudes. The latter, along with lack of understanding of the needs of those with DID, have resulted in services that offer inadequate supports and inequitable health and social care (12–14).

The experience of absence of a voice in daily circumstances affecting their lives is captured in more recent self-advocacy mantras such as 'Nothing about us without us' and 'Being with rather than doing to'. Taking the time to include patients with DID in all aspects of their assessment and care, and finding ways 'to listen' to their communication in whatever way this is being offered (e.g. interviewing in settings familiar to them, informal observations, paying special attention to body language in individuals without speech, careful history-taking involving informants who know the individual well), often illuminates the causes of their mental distress in ways that are not possible by simply applying criteria developed for a population without such disabilities (15). Adjustment problems may become chronic disorders in health or social care systems unwilling to learn directly from patients with DID or make the necessary accommodations to lessen their mental distress (16). Where more positive attitudes towards disabilities prevail, and necessary accommodations are made, communication, coping, and mental wellbeing are enhanced, and the impact of stressors diminished.

Personal profiles

Those with DID are characterized by heterogeneity of circumstances across multiple domains. In particular, each affected individual has a unique psychological and personal profile that needs to be considered in identifying the impact of, and response to, potential stressors, and assessing coping capacity. People with DID demonstrate a range of adaptive, cognitive, and communication capacities and skills. Different aetiologies (e.g. genetic [fragile X], environmental [FASD] (fetal alcohol spectrum disorders)) give rise to different physical and mental health vulnerabilities as well as different psychological and behavioural profiles (i.e. physical and behavioural phenotypes). Additionally, several conditions may coexist (e.g. medical conditions and disabilities such as epilepsy, cerebral palsy, and hearing or vision problems; unrecognized pain; coexisting psychiatric disorders; other early-onset developmental concerns such as autism spectrum disorder (ASD) (with sensory hypersensitivities), and ADHD (attention deficit hyperactivity disorder)) (17). Any or a combination of these circumstances will impact on activities of daily living, access to necessary supports, and mental wellbeing, especially at times of adjustment vulnerability such as transitions. Mismatch between individual needs and available networks of supports will give rise to ongoing stress, and less capacity or resilience to cope with, and adjust to, new demands.

Communication and cognitive difficulties may affect emotional development, and in particular, capacity to handle stress. Insecure attachment may be more common because of the psychological impact on parents and families of the news of difference/disability, or because of perceived unresponsiveness of the infant. Early life events may disrupt bonding and the experience of a secure base (e.g. negative life events associated with medical conditions such as hospital admissions or painful procedures); early separations may occur consequent to needed family respite; and inadequate financial, physical, and psychological supports for the family deplete care providers' emotional resources for the child. Some disabilities, associated with the unique needs of the child (e.g. coexisting DID, autism, sensory sensitivities, severe behavioural distress and 'meltdowns'), can place great demand on families and challenge services. While emotional difficulties and low-threshold negative responses to stressors may be managed adequately when the child is small (e.g. familiar adult to help regulate the emotional distress with physical comforting), this becomes more problematic as the child grows older and increases in size, and the care provider may be less familiar.

Typically-developing children start to acquire more independent strategies to manage stress and negative feelings with the emergence of imagination and language (e.g. by using words and stories). These strategies may develop later in individuals with DID who do develop language or some speech, but will not be available to those with more severe or profound DID, necessitating different strategies to help them cope. Ways to help a child or adult with severe or profound DID share feelings and wishes requires patience, imagination, and creativity. While more able individuals with DID may be able to learn to initiate effective coping strategies independently, for others the focus is on helping them seek the assistance of others at the times of upset (e.g. by use of a picture board or a red flash card). Those with the most profound disabilities may rely entirely on others to recognize their distress and provide a safe place and emotional support (18–22).

Stressors

Stressors are ubiquitous and multiple in the lives of people with DID, and negative life events, including harassment and abuse, are increased compared to events that occur within the general population (10,11,23). Stressors may be chronic (e.g. living settings and housemates not of their choice) and/or unpredictable (e.g. life events, such as carer illness or new staff unfamiliar with the individual), or occur as part of daily demands and expectations. Even small changes in usual day-to-day routines may be experienced as extremely stressful for some (see Box 10.1). Predictable psycho-social milestones give rise to developmental challenges (see Table 10.2) which, depending on the strengths and vulnerabilities of the individual involved, can present

Box 10.1 Sue: A case of recurrent adjustment disorder

A 17-year-old woman with autism, in the month before graduating from high school, started to engage in repetitive motor movements (e.g. repetitively touching walls, licking behaviours, expiratory exhalations), and at times would get 'stuck' and be unable to proceed further in any activity. Over the next few weeks, between occasions of getting stuck, her motor movements became more agitated; she would pinch herself, causing bruises, would scream intermittently for long periods, and had difficulty settling at night (running up and down stairs insisting she had to complete her laundry). Over the next few months she presented to the emergency department on several occasions and was treated symptomatically with trials of several anxiolytic and sedative medications, without benefit.

When referred to the specialist DID mental health team at age 20, she had experienced several such episodes, lasting several days to several months. Sometimes, symptoms of frenzied activity and anxiety were most notable; at other times she lost interest in usual pleasurable activities and had sleep disturbance and some weight loss. Over time, it became apparent that these episodic escalations occurred in relation to the following stressors, occurring individually or in combination: (a) medical issues—allergies, menses, constipation, (b) sensory hypersensitivities, e.g. certain smells, (c) ongoing intrusiveness of peers, (d) perceiving care provider stress, and (e) extreme difficulties in managing predictable, unpredictable events. For example, after establishing her routine of travelling in the van to her workplace, her behaviour suddenly deteriorated. The stressor was identified as a change in the van driver's routine so as to pick up other students. Her behaviour returned to usual baseline when she was informed, on getting into the van each morning, how many stops it would be before she arrived at her destination; this was supported by a social story that she would go over with staff the night before.

When specific accommodations were made for her autism, e.g. care providers being mindful of her sensory hypersensitivities and

Box 10.1 (Continued)

the need to self-regulate with deep pressure (such as a sensory mat) and motor activities (such as brushing her hair), the intensity of her behavioural and emotional responses, when these occurred, was lessened, and the responses were less prolonged too.

These episodes met the criteria for adjustment disorder (DSM- 5); the symptom pattern constituted a mix of anxiety and depressed mood (F309.28) and mixed disturbance of emotions and conduct (F309.4).

© Bradley, 2016

new adaptational opportunities or can precipitate a developmental crisis. In societies with highly developed habilitative (educational, vocational, and residential) systems, there may be predictable stressors owing to the nature of the system, and to transitions within it (see Table 10.3). Stressors involving negative interpersonal relationships seem to be a particular issue for people with disability (24-26).

Coping

People with DID thus develop along a path of atypical juxtaposition of biological, psychological, and social milestones (29). As well as differences in cognitive, adaptive, and communication skills and stages of emotional development, differences in executive functioning (30) and problem-solving strategies are described (24, 31). All contribute to difficulties in coping with situations that call for novel responses and increased autonomous functioning. The individual may respond to these stressors with recognizable signs of increased anxiety or may present with sudden, unpredictable aggression (even to skilled staff who are, however, unfamiliar with this individual), self-injury, non-compliance with some externally determined need, or withdrawal or regression from previous levels of autonomous functioning (16, 32, 33). These severe reactions may be in response to a stressor(s) so overwhelming, from the individual's perspective, that it is experienced as if life threatening, resulting in panic reactions and

Table 10.2 Predictable crises in the lives of people with DID[1]

Note: the crises listed in the left-hand column are explored in the Books Beyond Words (BBW)[2] series titles in the right-hand column

Crisis[3]	Supporting titles from the BBW series
Initial diagnosis of DID	
Birth of siblings	*Sonia's Feeling Sad*
Starting school/college	
Puberty and adolescence	*Susan's Growing Up; George Gets Smart*
Sex and dating	*Falling in Love; Loving Each Other Safely*
Being surpassed by younger siblings	*Michelle Finds a Voice*
Emancipation of siblings	*Sonia's Feeling Sad*
End of education	*George Gets Smart; Speaking Up for Myself*
Out-of-home placement/residential moves	*A New Home in the Community; Finding a Safe Place from Abuse; Ann has Dementia*
Staff/individual relationships	*Feeling Cross and Sorting It Out; Enjoying Sport and Exercise; The Drama Group*
Inappropriate expectation	*Hug Me, Touch Me; Making Friends*
Ageing, illness, death of parents	*When Mum Died; When Dad Died*
Death of peers, loss of friends	*When Somebody Dies*
Medical illness/psychiatric illness	*Getting on with Cancer; Ron's Feeling Blue; Getting on with Type 1 Diabetes; Getting on with Type 2 Diabetes; Getting on with Epilepsy; Looking After My Heart; Am I Going to Die?*
Deinstitutionalization	*A New Home in the Community; Peter's New Home*
Traumatic events	*Jenny Speaks Out; Bob Tells All; Mugged; When Dad Hurts Mum; I Can Get Through It; You're Under Arrest*

[1] from Levitas and Gilson (2001) (27)

[2] Hollins (28)

[3] For individuals with DID and/or family depending on age

© Bradley, Hollins, Korossy, Levitas, 2018

Table 10.3 Life events with negative impact

Events most commonly rated by adults with DID (%) as having negative impact[a] and links to *Books Beyond Words* (BBW) http://booksbeyondwords. co.uk/ [b] (or search for appropriate scenarios in the *Beyond Words* story app)

Event	%	BBW title
Permanent change in staffing	35	*A New Home in the Community, Ann has Dementia*
Other person moved into or out of house/flat/unit	24	*Jenny Speaks Out*
Period of cover by non-regular carer	22	*Feeling Cross and Sorting It Out*
Serious illness or injury not requiring hospitalization	19	*Going to the Doctor; Am I Going to Die?*
Separation from friend/family/long-term carer	16	*A New Home in the Community*
Moved house	13	*Peter's New Home*
Change in daily routine	12	*George Gets Smart*
Subjected to verbal abuse (bullying)	12	*Speaking Up for Myself; Finding a Safe Place from Abuse; Making Friends; Hug Me, Touch Me*
Witnessed physical attack or verbal abuse of another	12	*When Dad Hurts Mum*
Moved room, change in decoration/furniture	10	*Jenny Speaks Out; Peter's New Home*
Victim of violence	10	*Supporting Victims; Mugged; Finding a Safe Place from Abuse*
Introduction/change/withdrawal of medication	7	*Ron's Feeling Blue; Sonia's Feeling Sad; Getting on with Epilepsy*

[a] From Hulbert-Williams 2014 (23)

[b] Hollins (28)

© Bradley, Holline, Korossy, Levitas, 2018

activation of instinctive survival responses such as Fight (aggression to self, to others, and to the environment)—Flight (running away)—Freeze (catatonic-like movements) and immobilization (32, 34). However, with careful planning, support, and skill development, potential stressors become opportunities for successful developmental attainment (29, 35).

Adjustment disorder diagnosis

If unrecognized, responses to these-day-to-day and developmental challenges can lead to AD, as well as post-traumatic stress disorder (PTSD) or other major psychiatric disorders. Adjustment disorders have been reconceptualized in DSM-5 under 'Trauma and Stressor-Related Disorders' (along with acute stress disorder, post-traumatic stress disorder, and reactive attachment and disinhibited social engagement disorders), a group of disorders described as a heterogeneous array of stress–response syndromes that occur after exposure to a distressing (traumatic or non-traumatic) circumstance; subtypes are marked by differences in mood, anxiety, emotions, and conduct.

Diagnostic criteria for AD are conceptually similar in both DSM-5 and ICD-10, with some differences occurring in relation to the timing of onset and duration of disorder in relation to the stressor event. Criteria for DSM-5 and ICD-10 adjustment disorders and key adaptations made for people with DID (DM-ID & DC-LD) are outlined in Table 10.1.

Barriers to diagnosing adjustment disorders in those with DID

The nature of the lives of people with DID

Clinicians unfamiliar with the lives of people with DID may not appreciate the impact of some stressors (e.g. the death of a parent may have been compounded by the bereaved person also losing a home, familiar routines, and primary confidante). Clinicians may not fully understand that difficulties with accessing services, or lack of adequate supports, may lead to diminished coping ability and escalating frustrations. Instead, they may consider the presenting symptoms and behaviours as 'problem' behaviours or symptoms of major psychiatric disorder requiring treatment—rather than a consequence of circumstances which require careful scrutiny to determine needed services and engagement in tenacious advocacy to meet these requirements (16). Other diagnoses that fail to recognize relevant context include 'oppositional defiant disorder' in individuals who have never had the opportunity or ability to develop non-behavioural means of mediating or communicating distress, and 'intermittent explosive disorder' to describe behaviours that are, in fact, behavioural reactions to identifiable stressors.

The nature of stressors

Identification

For adults with DID living away from the family home, it is often very difficult to elicit a pre-morbid or immediate past history to identify ongoing stressors or specific triggers to the presenting mental distress. Incomplete histories arise where there are discontinuities in care and quick turnover of care staff (both circumstances also being potential stressors), problems with obtaining consent, difficulties in sharing information across health and social care systems and differences in the length of time historical information is kept. Informants who do not know the individual well may provide unreliable information.

Stressors may be hidden by a defensive care system where past abuses occurred, surfacing only as behavioural responses to triggers in current daily living and described as 'out of the blue' behaviours by care providers until better understood in the context of the past abuse (36-38). For example, the report of a woman who screamed several times a day until observation of her immediate environment linked her screaming to the sound of running water and a boiling kettle. Her direct support staff were unaware that she had been burnt by boiling water from a kettle in a previous placement—the screaming stopped when the triggers were removed (39).

The chronic nature of some stressors can serve to conceal them; they might be thought of as inherent rather than modifiable factors in a person's life.

Stressors associated with the cause of the DID may not be understood by care providers. For example, some developmental conditions are associated with neurobiological circumstances that result in different sensory and perceptual experiences (such as sensory hypersensitivities in autism). Environments considered adequate or even pleasing to care providers may be experienced as extremely distressing for those with autism. Care providers may fail to appreciate how painful these environments can be from an autism perspective (as in Sue's case; see Box 10.1).

Timing of stressors

Criteria for AD include onset of symptoms within 1 month (ICD-10) to 3 months (DSM-5) following the stressor. Symptoms should not persist for longer than 6 months after the cessation of the stressor or its consequences (note: one exception to this in ICD-10 is 'prolonged depressive reaction that should not exceed 2 yrs'; in DSM-IV-TR there is a specifier for when the disturbance lasts longer than 6 months—see Table 10.1).

To meet these criteria requires both identification of the stressor and resolution or removal of the stressor. Because stressors are not always obvious to care providers or clinicians, they may continue for years. In clinical practice, when there is a history of sudden onset of mental distress or significant change in behaviour, it is essential to screen for the occurrence of any significant events (even those that might be considered positive—such as Christmas; see Box 10.2) (40), change in life circumstances, or other potential stressors in the individual's current, recent, or past history. For long-standing mental distress and behaviours that challenge, identifying the first onset of concerns and detailing events around this time, as for sudden onset, often prove to be rewarding in terms of identifying stressors. This may require scrutinizing past medical and hospital records and reviewing past personal history with family and others. Careful observation of 'problem' behaviours and their antecedents may alert clinicians and care providers to uniquely experienced stressors (e.g. acting out behaviours, refusal, non-compliance, and running behaviours that may present in some environments but not in others, and as such point to stressful circumstances in the environment in which they occur) (41). If the stressor is not identified, there is risk of a mental disorder other than AD being diagnosed.

Challenges in diagnosing psychiatric disorders in those with DID

Clinicians may lack experience in appreciating the signs of anxiety and depression in people with DID (42–44). Coexisting ASD complicates the assessment of anxiety (32, 45–47). In general psychiatry, mood state in AD has been described as depending on the cognitive presence of the stressor compared to the diurnal change or reduced mood

Box 10.2 Complexities in identifying stressors and diagnosing adjustment (and other psychiatric) disorders in people with DID

In this study, episodic (e.g. mood) and non-episodic (e.g. ADHD, tics, phobias, compulsive) (48, 49) disorders were explored separately. 'Circumscribed episodic disorders' were identified associated with adverse circumstances, such as a change in care arrangements or schooling, and seemed to resolve when the change was reversed and care arrangements were improved. The symptoms were not sufficiently distinct to warrant a specific diagnosis. It seemed likely that these disorders were forms of adjustment disorder as conceptualized in DSM-IV (American Psychiatric Association, 1994), but this diagnostic category did exist in Research Diagnostic

Criteria (Endicott & Spitzer, 1978; Spitzer et al, 1978) for major psychiatric disorders. Moreover, there was some lack of clarity over the precise timing of the interrelationship between the stressor and the onset and offset of the episodic disorders, so it remained unclear whether all of these symptoms represented adjustment phenomena.

Except for one individual in the autism group, these were single-episode disorders. Identified stressors were similar for both groups, and included lack of understanding of needs in the school setting, transition to high school and inadequate supports, and physical and sexual abuse at home and at school. One individual with autism suffered an episode of illness (AD) with the approach of Christmas each year, and a further episode when his mother was unable to provide the usual level of support because of her own mental health problems.

These circumscribed episodes were characterized by challenging behaviours. The adverse circumstances giving rise to such behaviours were not always immediately obvious to the care providers, and often came to be understood as relevant only after the circumstance was no longer present.

The higher prevalence of both episodic and non-episodic disorders, and overlapping disorders in individuals with ASD

(*continued*)

Box 10.2 (Continued)

and DID, compared to the prevalence of these in those with ID-only, highlighted the importance of: (a) carefully establishing individual baseline (pre-morbid) functioning and behaviours when conducting psychiatric assessments of people with DID, and (b) screening for unique biopsychosocial vulnerabilities and triggers to the individuals' mental distress.

Source: data from Br J Psychiatry, **189**(4), Bradley E, Bolton P, Episodic psychiatric disorders in teenagers with learning disabilities with and without autism, pp. 361–366, Copyright (2006), Royal College of Psychiatrists

reactivity in a major depressive episode (50). However, for those with DID, this distinction may be less easily determined or obvious in clinical practice—a reminder to the clinician of the necessity to establish the patient's unique baseline (pre-morbid) mood and functioning as a preliminary to the psychiatric evaluation (40). Additionally, the chronic nature of stressors can confound the diagnosis of another psychiatric disorder as well as the development of a superimposed AD. In people with ASD, AD may present as panic episodes, or rather, they have panic disorder, exacerbated by acute stressors, perhaps justifying both diagnoses. Mechanistic application of standard psychiatric criteria, and mental health or behavioural checklists, will miss the contextual features of AD and its correct diagnosis.

Bereavement

Normal bereavement reactions are not considered an AD. However, where anger and irritability and resulting disturbance of conduct occur, AD diagnosis with disturbance of conduct or with mixed disturbance of emotion and conduct is warranted in DM-ID (see Box 10.3). Bereavement may be experienced in response to a variety of losses: death of close family members, friends, or pets; separations and departures consequent to staff changes, promotions, and retirements; or changes in residence, daily activities, and routines (see Tables 10.2 and 10.3). The expression of grief may be confounded by being delayed. One of the authors recalls a gentleman who started to kick the family dog and to destroy his most treasured possessions at around the time of the first

Box 10.3 Sam: A case of adjustment disorder with mixed anxiety and conduct problem

A 40-year-old man with mild DID was brought by police to the emergency department (ED) after he smashed a candy machine on a nearby subway platform. He could only scream, 'The candle, I saw the candle in the jar'. It became clear that he'd been referring to a Yahrzeit candle, a Jewish commemoration of the anniversary of the death of a parent. When reassured he was not in legal trouble, he calmed to the extent of being able to give the contact information of the sister he lived with. He calmed further when she arrived, and the following story emerged.

He had lived with his sister for the year since his mother's death, and had been able to keep to his long-accustomed routine. This was the first anniversary of the death, and he and his sister were anticipating the unveiling ceremony, when the memorial stone is 'unveiled'. As this event approached, he had become increasingly anxious, to the point of disturbed sleep and tearfulness and anger at any perceived disapproval. On the morning of the Emergence room visit, he followed his usual routine: he packed his lunch and the exact amount of money he needed for his train fare, and for the snack he would buy.

That morning, however, he was anxious, and tried to buy the snack at the candy machine on the subway platform. The machine was broken, and when no candy came out he put in another coin. The machine again failed, and he panicked at the thought that he now had less than he needed for his return train fare, 'and I couldn't get home from the workshop'. He began hitting at the machine, hoping to get his money back. He smashed the machine's mirror front and was then approached by a passing police officer. Recognizing a mental disability of some kind, and his degree of distress, the police officer took him to the emergency department rather than the police station.

He was able to go home with his sister, with the promise of follow-up psychotherapy.

© Levitas, 2016

anniversary of his mother's death—nobody had spoken about it, nobody thought that he had been distressed by the death, and nobody made a connection between his changed behaviour and his mother's death.

Assessment and diagnosis

When mental health and behavioural concerns arise, a multi-perspective biopsychosocial approach is recommended to identify potential stressors present in the broad range of circumstances in the lives of people with DID (2, 51, 52). Medical conditions, supports, and environments inadequate in individual circumstances, expectations inappropriate to developmental achievements, and past unresolved trauma all need to be considered as potential contributing factors, and comprehensively explored (53, 54). Coexisting psychiatric conditions may also contribute to vulnerability to stress and require systematic identification (see Box 10.2). Identifying specific triggers, assessment of stress, and screening for adjustment-related issues is crucial. Major psychiatric disorder must be actively sought for in the diagnostic process as well as ruled out. For example, AD with depressed mood is quite different and a considerably more favourable diagnosis than major depressive disorder. Familiarity with circumstances that can precipitate a crisis in the lives of people with DID, along with a timely mental health consultation, can result in accurate diagnosis and more rapid therapeutic resolution (see Tables 10.2 and 10.3).

The following instruments are available to assess psycho-social stresses specifically for people with intellectual disability (55):

The *Lifestress Inventory for Adults with Intellectual Disability* (25) is an interview schedule for individuals who can respond to the questions; an informant version is also available (26).

The *Stress Survey Schedule for Individuals with Autism and Other Pervasive Developmental Disabilities* (56) describes situations commonly experienced as stressful by persons with ASD, e.g. 'receiving hugs and affection' or 'waiting in line'. Informant and self-report versions are evaluated (56, 57).

Prevalence of adjustment disorder in DID

Research on AD in DID is limited (58). A literature review by the current authors identified only one population-based clinical evaluation study of mental health disorders in adults with DID that included this disorder (59). This study is also unique in providing comparison between clinical, DC-LD, ICD-10-DCR, and DSM-IV-TR diagnostic criteria. Considerably lower prevalence rates using ICD-10-DCR and DSM-IV-TR diagnostic criteria were found, highlighting the importance of taking into consideration developmental level in understanding psychopathology within categories of mental disorders (59). The point prevalence rate of mental ill-health (clinical diagnoses) was 40.9%—and 28.3% when problem behaviours were excluded. Mental ill-health was associated with more life events, type of support, lower ability, and more consultations with the family doctor in the previous 12 months. The point prevalence (clinical diagnoses) of anxiety disorders was 3.8%, with AD and PTSD showing similar rates (0.5% and 0.3%, respectively).

Using the Psychopathology Inventory for Mentally Retarded Adults, which has subscales for 'Adjustment Disorder' and 'Inappropriate Adjustment', Gustafsson et al. (60) identified mental health problems in samples from two Swedish counties. The percentage of individuals above the cut-off point was highest for 'Anxiety Disorder' (26.8%), followed by 'Inappropriate Adjustment' (27.5%) and 'AD' (21.1%).

Bakken et al. (61) reported on general and severe adjustment problems (GAPs and SGAPs, respectively), as well as four psychiatric disorders—psychosis, depression, anxiety, and obsessive-compulsive disorder (OCD)—in two groups with DID—one with ASD, and one without. Psychiatric disorders and SGAPs were found to be high in both the ASD group (53.2%) and DID-only group (17.4%); more than 50% of the ASD group, and approximately 20% of the DID-only group, had SGAPs. The authors conclude that having DID seems to imply high risk for developing adjustment problems, and that it is especially difficult for those with ASD to master everyday challenges.

In one population-based study of teenagers identified with DID, those with DID and autism were matched on age, gender, and nonverbal IQ to those with DID only (40). A semi-structured, psychiatric, informant-based assessment was conducted for all participants to identify episodic disorders (e.g. mood), with separate schedules used to identify background (i.e. non-episodic) conditions (e.g. ADHD, OCD). While not specifically looking for adjustment disorder (as this category did not exist in the research diagnostic criteria used in the study), the clinical circumstances suggesting AD were compelling for several participants (see Box 10.2). These findings confirm the complexities in the presentation of mental distress in DID and ASD and the benefits of distinguishing episodes of mental disorder from background disorders. The findings also illuminated how attempts to standardize clinical criteria for research purposes may inadvertently exclude clinical phenomena that require evaluation by an experienced clinician.

Several studies have examined AD in clinical samples:

Eight per cent of adults attending a specialist DID mental health service were diagnosed with AD (62).

A retrospective outpatient chart review of patients with DID matched to non-DID patients found rates of AD at 1% (mild) and 2% (moderate to profound) in those with DID, compared to 2% in the non-DID group (63).

Raitasuo et al. (64) studied the demographic, medical, and psychosocial characteristics of individuals with DID referred for inpatient admission and matched on age, gender, and functioning level to non-psychiatric-disorder DID individuals. At discharge, 22% with DID were diagnosed with AD.

Finally, Levitas (65) found a rate of 3% with AD in a 2,144 DID patient database of the Division of Prevention and Treatment of Developmental Disorders, Stratford, New Jersey, USA.

Treatment

Removal of the stressor

Even if identified, care systems may not recognize a particular circumstance as being overly stressful and beyond the individual's coping capacity. For example, hypersensitivities may be experienced as extremely painful by someone with ASD. Care systems may focus on trying to change the individual's behavioural response ('problem behaviours') rather than taking measures to reduce the sensory discomfort—or conclude that it is the individual who should adapt, especially if removing the stressor places further demand on scarce resources. Assisting service systems and care providers to understand the link between the stressor and the diagnosed individual's response in the context of his/her particular vulnerabilities is an important part of treatment. Ideally, the treating clinician should advocate for removal of the stressor rather than giving way to requests for medication to manage stressor-related behaviours and the risk of chronic adjustment disorder.

Psychotherapy

Psychotherapy and/or counselling is considered the mainstay of treatment for AD in the general population, minimizing the emotional impact of the stressor and enhancing coping if the stressor cannot be removed or reduced (66).

Several psychological approaches shown to be helpful in the general population (66) have been successfully adapted for people with DID (67). Pictures and stories created specifically for therapeutic use when working with older children and adults with DID are now available (28, 68). Reading wordless books one to one, in group therapy and in community book clubs, helps individuals with DID to re-frame their own stories and empowers them with new coping mechanisms (see Tables 10.2 and 10.3) (69, 70). The ability to self-regulate emotions is critical to their health and wellbeing (70).

For those with more limited communication (severe to profound DID), emotional reassurance and affect regulation are enhanced by individuals being supported in familiar routines, in familiar environments with familiar care providers. For individuals with limited or no language skills, approaches that use body language to engage emotionally have been found to be effective in reducing behavioural distress (71-74).

Successful treatment benefits from the different aspects of the individual's support system working collaboratively to maximize adaptation (75). Supportive scaffolding around the individual may need to be increased until coping and functioning return to pre-stressor baselines.

Pharmacotherapy

Pharmacotherapy may be used for concomitant mood (e.g. depression, anxiety) (66) symptoms.

Prevention

Care providers can be supported to proactively identify circumstances that are likely to be stressful to the individuals they are supporting (see Tables 10.2 and 10.3), as well as individual/specific concerns (e.g. hypersensitivities in autism, past history of trauma) and concerns about retraumatization. Identifying potential stressor(s) offers opportunities to prepare for transitions and prevention. A range of psychological and behavioural therapies that enhance emotional resilience, affect regulation, and communication are now available to assist individuals with DID in day-to-day coping, managing stress (and trauma), building self-esteem, and increasing their personal sense of empowerment (67, 76, 77). People often understand pictures better than words. The Beyond Words approach tells stories about important or difficult events that happen to them in their lives. The pictures speak for themselves and they tell what could happen and show how people deal with their feelings. These books can be employed in preparation for an event (potential stressor), or therapeutically after the stressful event (see Tables 10.2 and 10.3).

Conclusion

For individuals with DID, challenges in everyday living contribute to greater vulnerability to psychiatric disorders and problem behaviours compared to their non-IDD peers (78). The prevalence of psychopathology is even greater when DID and autism coexist, the latter being a condition where change and transition are particularly difficult (79). Apart from individual developmental challenges, given the greater exposure to negative life events and adversity in this population, increased risk for stressor-related disorders such as AD might be expected (23, 80, 81).

However, there are perplexing issues yet to be fully elucidated in clinical research. Symptoms of AD overlap with problem behaviours (5), and problem behaviours and anxiety are associated (82). Life events are associated with affective and neurotic problems, anger, and aggression (23). Indicators of adjustment problems are often observed in individuals with DID and psychiatric disorders (45, 61, 83). The relationship between psychiatric disorders and problem behaviours in DID remains unclear (38, 84, 85). Added to this complexity are findings that signs of physiological arousal may be difficult to recognize when autism and DID coexist (32).

In the absence of an identified stressor, an AD diagnosis cannot be made. Consequently, when a stressor is present but unrecognized (a common occurrence in DID), a disorder of mood, general anxiety, or problem behaviours may be diagnosed instead and treated accordingly. Mental distress may therefore be medicated, or a behavioural intervention put into effect, rather than the stressor being removed and psychological support offered (best practice). Additionally, if the (unrecognized) stressor remains, an AD may become chronic or recurrent and may then be perceived as a 'treatment-resistant' psychiatric disorder.

In general psychiatric practice, the gold standard for AD diagnosis is the trained clinician (86, 87); in DID services, the latter must be someone knowledgeable about the lives of people with DID. In the clinical setting, routinely screening for stressors (including detailed interviews with family carers about past experiences), and ruling out AD before making a more serious psychiatric diagnosis, should (a) improve diagnostic accuracy, (b) offer opportunity for more immediate relief from mental distress, and (c) reduce the risk of inappropriate use of psychotropic medication (88) or behavioural interventions which have failed to eliminate a continuing stressor.

References

1. **World Health Organization**. The ICD-10 classification of mental and behavioural disorders: Diagnostic criteria for research. Geneva: World Health Organization; 1993.

2. **Royal College of Psychiatrists**. DC-LD: Diagnostic criteria for psychiatric disorders for use with adults with learning disabilities/mental retardation. London: Gaskell; 2001.

3. **American Psychiatric Association**. Diagnostic and statistical manual of mental disorders DSM-IV-TR. 4th ed. Washington, DC: American Psychiatric Association; 2000.

4. **Fletcher R, Loschen E, Stavrakaki C, First M**, editors. DM-ID: Diagnostic manual—intellectual disability: A textbook of diagnosis of mental disorders in persons with intellectual disability. Kingston, NY: National Association for the Dually Diagnosed (NADD); 2007.

5. **Levitas A, Hurley AD.** Adjustment disorders. In: Fletcher R, Loschen E, Stavrakaki C, First M, editors. Diagnostic manual—intellectual disability: A textbook of diagnosis of mental disorders in persons with intellectual disability. Kingston, NY: National Association for the Dually Diagnosed; 2007. p. 497–510.

6. **American Psychiatric Association.** Diagnostic and statistical manual of mental disorders: DSM-5. 5th ed. Arlington, VA: American Psychiatric Association; 2013.

7. **Banks R, Bush A, Baker P, Bradshaw J, Carpenter P, Deb S,** et al. Challenging behaviour: a unified approach. College Report CR144. 2007; Retrieved 31 March 2016 from: http://www.rcpsych.ac.uk/files/pdfversion/cr144.pdf, accessed 25 October 2017.

8. **Banks R, Bush A;** Other Contributors. Challenging behaviour: a unified approach—update: Clinical and service guidelines for supporting children, young people and adults with intellectual disabilities who are at risk of receiving abusive or restrictive practices. Faculty Report FR/ID/08. 2016; Retrieved 25 April 2016 from: www.rcpsych.ac.uk/pdf/FR_ID_08.pdf, accessed 25 October 2017.

9. **Brown I, Radford JP.** Historical overview of intellectual and developmental disabilities. In: Brown I, Percy M, editors. A comprehensive guide to intellectual and developmental disabilities. Baltimore, MD: Paul H. Brookes, Publishing; 2007. p. 17–33.

10. **Beadle-Brown J, Richardson L, Guest C, Malovic A, Bradshaw J, Himmerich J.** Living in fear: Better outcomes for people with learning disabilities and autism. Main research report. Canterbury: Tizard Centre, University of Kent; 2014. Retrieved July 2016 from: http://www.mcch.org.uk/pages/multimedia/db_document.document?id=8009, accessed 25 October 2017.

11. **Gravell C.** Loneliness & cruelty: People with learning disability and their experience of harassment, abuse and related crime in the community. London, UK: Lemos and Crane; 2012. Retrieved 12 July 2016 from: http://www.lemosandcrane.co.uk/home/resources/loneliness.pdf, accessed 25 October 2017.

12. **Tuffrey-Wijne I, Giatras N, Goulding L, Abraham E, Fenwick L, Edwards C,** et al. Identifying the factors affecting the implementation of strategies to promote a safer environment for patients with learning disabilities in NHS hospitals: a mixed-methods study. HS&DR. 2013;**1**(13).

13. **Tuffrey-Wijne I, Hollins S.** Preventing 'deaths by indifference': identification of reasonable adjustments is key. Br J Psychiatry. 2014;**205**(2):86–87.

14. **Heslop P, Blair P, Fleming P, Hoghton M, Marriott A, Russ L.** Confidential Inquiry into premature deaths of people with learning disabilities (CIPOLD). Final report, 2013. Retrieved from: http://www.bris.ac.uk/media-library/sites/cipold/migrated/documents/fullfinalreport.pdf, accessed 25 October 2017.

15. **Bradley E, Caldwell P, Korossy M.** 'Nothing about us without us': Understanding mental health and mental distress in individuals with

intellectual and developmental disabilities and autism through their inclusion, participation, and unique ways of communicating. Journal of Religion & Society, Supplement Series. 2015(suppl 12):94–109. Available from: https://dspace.creighton.edu/xmlui/bitstream/handle/10504/65683/2015-32.pdf?sequence=3, accessed 25 October 2017.

16. Palucka AM, Reid M, Holstein A. The clinical profiles of women with intellectual disabilities and affective or adjustment disorder utilizing mental health services. J Dev Disabl. 2010;**16**(1):12–17.

17. Cooper SA, McLean G, Guthrie B, McConnachie A, Mercer S, Sullivan F, et al. Multiple physical and mental health comorbidity in adults with intellectual disabilities: population-based cross-sectional analysis. BMC Fam Pract. 2015;**16**:110.

18. Tuffrey-Wijne I, Hollins S, Curfs L. Supporting patients who have intellectual disabilities: a survey investigating staff training needs. Int J Palliat Nurs. 2005;**11**(4):182–8.

19. Caldwell P, Horwood J. From isolation to intimacy: Making friends without words. London; Philadelphia: Jessica Kingsley; 2007.

20. Caldwell P. Delicious conversations: Reflections on autism, intimacy and communication. Brighton, UK: Pavilion Press; 2012.

21. Regnard C, Matthews D, Gibson L, Learning Disability and Palliative Care Team at Northgate Hospital in Northumberland, UK. DisDAT: Disability Distress Assessment Tool (DisDat). v20; Retrieved Jul 20, 2016 from: http://www.stoswaldsuk.org/how-we-help/we-educate/resources/disdat.aspx.

22. Regnard C, Reynolds J, Watson B, Matthews D, Gibson L, Clarke C. Understanding distress in people with severe communication difficulties: developing and assessing the Disability Distress Assessment Tool (DisDAT). J Intellect Disabil Res. 2007;**51**(4):277–92.

23. Hulbert-Williams L, Hastings R, Owen DM, Burns L, Day J, Mulligan J, et al. Exposure to life events as a risk factor for psychological problems in adults with intellectual disabilities: a longitudinal design. J Intellect Disabil Res. 2014;**58**(1):48–60.

24. Hartley SL, MacLean WE Jr. Depression in adults with mild intellectual disability: Role of stress, attributions, and coping. Am J Intellect Dev Disabil 2009;**114**(3):147–160.

25. Bramston P, Fogarty G, Cummins RA. The nature of stressors reported by people with an intellectual disability. J Appl Res Intellect Disabil. 1999;**12**(1):1–10.

26. Lunsky Y, Bramston P. A preliminary study of perceived stress in adults with intellectual disabilities according to self-report and informant ratings. J Intellect Dev Disabil. 2006;**31**(1):20–27.

27. Levitas AS, Gilson SF. Predictable crises in the lives of people with mental retardation. Mental Health Aspects of Developmental Disabilities.

2001;**4**(3):89–100. Available from: http://media.wix.com/ugd//e11630_3dfd0a fd30344475d98cbffa253f6c92.pdf.

28. **Hollins S.** Books beyond words. 1989-2016; Available from: http://www. booksbeyondwords.co.uk/welcome.

29. **Levitas A, Gilson SF.** Psychosocial development of children and adolescents with mild mental retardation. In: Bouras N, editor. Mental health in mental retardation: Recent advances and practices. Cambridge, UK; New York: Cambridge University Press; 1994. p. 34–45.

30. **Janke K, Klein-Tasman B.** Executive functions in intellectual disability syndromes. In: Hunter SJ, Sparrow EP, editors. Executive function and dysfunction: Identification, assessment, and treatment. Cambridge; New York: Cambridge University Press; 2012. p. 109–22.

31. **Hartley SL, Maclean WE.** Coping strategies of adults with mild intellectual disability for stressful social interactions. J Ment Health Res Intellect Disabil. 2008;**1**(2):109–27.

32. **Helverschou SB, Martinsen H.** Anxiety in people diagnosed with autism and intellectual disability: recognition and phenomenology. Res Autism Spectr Disord. 2011;**5**(1):377–87.

33. **Loos HG, Loos Miller IM.** Shutdown states and stress instability in autism. 2004; Retrieved Mar 15, 2016 from: http://www.de-poort.be/cgi-bin/ Document.pl?id=374.

34. **Loos Miller IM, Loos HG.** Shutdowns and stress in autism. 2004; Retrieved July 30, 2016 from: https://autismawarenesscentre.com/shutdowns-stress-autism/.

35. **Levitas A, Hurley AD.** Diagnosis and treatment of adjustment disorders in people with intellectual disability. Mental Health Aspects of Developmental Disabilities. 2005;**8**(2):52–60.

36. **Hubert J, Hollins S.** Men with severe learning disabilities and challenging behaviour in long-stay hospital care: qualitative study. Br J Psychiatry. 2006;**188**:70–4.

37. **Sequeira H, Hollins S.** Clinical effects of sexual abuse on people with learning disability: critical literature review. Br J Psychiatry. 2003;**182**:13–19.

38. **Sequeira H, Howlin P, Hollins S.** Psychological disturbance associated with sexual abuse in people with learning disabilities. Case-control study. Br J Psychiatry. 2003;**183**:451–6.

39. **Ryan R.** Posttraumatic stress disorder in persons with developmental disabilities. Community Ment Health J. 1994;**30**(1):45–54.

40. **Bradley E, Bolton P.** Episodic psychiatric disorders in teenagers with learning disabilities with and without autism. Br J Psychiatry. 2006;**189**:361–6.

41. **Bradley E, Caldwell P.** Mental health and autism: Promoting Autism FaVourable Environments (PAVE). J Dev Disabl. 2013;**19**(1):8–23.

42. **Lunsky Y, Bradley E, Durbin J, Koegl C.** A comparison of patients with intellectual disability receiving specialised and general services in Ontario's psychiatric hospitals. J Intellect Disabil Res. 2008;**52**(11):1003–12.

43. **Palucka AM, Bradley E, Lunsky Y.** A case of unrecognized intellectual disability and autism misdiagnosed as schizophrenia: are there lessons to be learned? Mental Health Aspects of Developmental Disabilities. 2008;**11**(2):55–60.

44. **Edwards N, Lennox N, White P.** Queensland psychiatrists' attitudes and perceptions of adults with intellectual disability. J Intellect Disabil Res. 2007;**51**(Pt 1):75–81.

45. **Helverschou SB, Bakken TL, Martinsen H.** Identifying symptoms of psychiatric disorders in people with autism and intellectual disability: an empirical conceptual analysis. Mental Health Aspects of Developmental Disabilities. 2008;**11**(4):1–11.

46. **Cervantes PE, Matson JL.** Comorbid symptomology in adults with autism spectrum disorder and intellectual disability. J Autism Dev Disord. 2015;**45**(12):3961–70.

47. **Bradley E, Lunsky Y, Palucka A, Homitidis S.** Recognition of intellectual disabilities and autism in psychiatric inpatients diagnosed with schizophrenia and other psychotic disorders. Adv Ment Health Intellect Disabl. 2011;**5**(6):4–18.

48. **Bradley E, Ames C Bolton, P.** Psychiatric conditions and behavioural problems in adolescents with intellectual disabilities: correlates with autism. (2011). Canadian J Psychiatry. 2011; **56**(2):102–9.

49. **Bradley EA, Isaacs, BJ.** In attention, hyperactivity, and impulsivity in teenagers with intellectual disabilities, with and without autism. Canadian J Psychiatry. 2006;**51**(9):598–06.

50. **Baumeister H, Maercker A, Casey P.** Adjustment disorder with depressed mood: a critique of its DSM-IV and ICD-10 conceptualisations and recommendations for the future. Psychopathology. 2009;**42**(3):139–47.

51. **Charlot LR.** Chapter 132: Multidisciplinary assessment. In: **Rubin IL, Merrick J, Greydanus DE, Patel DR, editors.** Health care for people with intellectual and developmental disabilities across the lifespan. Rubin and Crocker 3rd ed. Springer; 2016. p. 1677–98.

52. **Holland A.** Chapter 1: Disorders of intellectual development: Historical, conceptual, epidemiological and nosological overview. In: **Woodbury-Smith M, editor.** Clinical topics in disorders of intellectual development. London, UK: Royal College of Psychiatrists Publications; 2015. p. 3–21.

53. **Lindsay P, Hoghton M.** Chapter 28: Practicalities of care for adults with intellectual and developmental disabilities. In: Rubin IL, Merrick J, Greydanus DE, Patel DR, editors. Health care for people with intellectual and developmental disabilities across the lifespan. Rubin and Crocker 3rd ed. Springer; 2016. p. 313–34.

54. **Bradley E, Korossy M.** Chapter 5: Behaviour problems. In: Woodbury-Smith M, editor. Clinical topics in disorders of intellectual development. London, UK: Royal College of Psychiatrists Publications; 2015. p. 72–112.

55. **Hurley AD, Levitas A, Luiselli JK, Moss S, Bradley E, Bailey N.** Chapter 2: Assessment and diagnostic procedure. In: Fletcher R, Cooper SA, Barnhill J, editors. Diagnostic manual—intellectual disability (DM-ID-2): A textbook of diagnosis of mental disorders in persons with intellectual disability. Kingston, NY: National Association for the Dually Diagnosed (NADD); 2017.

56. **Groden J, Diller A, Bausman M, Velicer W, Norman G, Cautela J.** The development of a stress survey schedule for persons with autism and other developmental disabilities. J Autism Dev Disord. 2001;**31**(2):207–17.

57. **Goodwin MS, Groden J, Velicer WF, Diller A.** Brief report: validating the stress survey schedule for persons with autism and other developmental disabilities. Focus Autism Other Dev Disabl. 2007;**22**(3):183–9.

58. **Dodd P, Kelly F.** Chapter 9: Stress, traumatic and bereavement reactions. In: Hemmings C, Bouras N, editors. Psychiatric and behavioral disorders in intellectual and developmental disabilities. 3rd ed. Cambridge, UK: Cambridge University Press; 2016. p. 99–108.

59. **Cooper SA, Smiley E, Morrison J, Williamson A, Allan L.** Mental ill-health in adults with intellectual disabilities: prevalence and associated factors. Br J Psychiatry. 2007;**190**:27–35.

60. **Gustafsson C, Sonnander K.** Occurrence of mental health problems in Swedish samples of adults with intellectual disabilities. Soc Psychiatry Psychiatr Epidemiol. 2004;**39**(6):448–56.

61. **Bakken TL, Helverschou SB, Eilertsen DE, Heggelund T, Myrbakk E, Martinsen H.** Psychiatric disorders in adolescents and adults with autism and intellectual disability: a representative study in one county in Norway. Res Dev Disabil. 2010;**31**(6):1669–77.

62. **Sturmey P, Newton J, Crowley A, Bouras N, Holt G.** The PAS-ADD Checklist: independent replication of its psychometric properties in a community sample. Br J Psychiatry 2005;**186**(4):319–23.

63. **Hurley AD, Folstein M, Lam N.** Patients with and without intellectual disability seeking outpatient psychiatric services: diagnoses and prescribing pattern. J Intellect Disabil Res. 2003;**47**(Pt 1):39–50.

64. **Raitasuo S, Taiminen T, Salokangas RK.** Characteristics of people with intellectual disability admitted for psychiatric inpatient treatment. J Intellect Disabil Res. 1999;**43**(Pt 2):112–18.

65. **Levitas A.** Survey of the first 2144 patients of the UMDNJ-SOM MH/ID Clinic. Unpublished data; [Data available upon request levitaan@rowan.edu].

66. **Strain JJ.** Chapter 4: Adjustment disorders: epidemiology, diagnosis and treatment. In: **Casey PR, Strain JJ,** editors. Trauma- and stressor-related disorders: A handbook for clinicians. Arlington, VA: American Psychiatric Association Publishing; 2016. p. 59–80.

67. **Beail N,** Faculties for Intellectual Disabilities of the Royal College of Psychiatrists and the Division of Clinical Psychology,British Psychological Society. Psychological therapies and people who have intellectual disabilities. 2016; Retrieved May 2, 2016 from: http://www.bps.org.uk/system/files/ Public%20files/Policy/psychological_therapies_and_people_who_have_id_ pdf_for_review.pdf.

68. **Bradley E, Hollins S.** Books Beyond Words: Using pictures to communicate. Journal on Developmental Disabilities 2013;**19**(1):24–32. Available from: http:// www.oadd.org/docs/41015_JoDD_19-1_24-32_Bradley_and_Hollins.pdf.

69. **Carmichael S.** How to start your own Beyond Words book club. 2016; Retrieved Aug 1, 2016 from: http://static1.squarespace.com/static/ 551cfff9e4b0f74d74cb307e/t/56444e98e4b014f5dbb566e6/1447317144514/ BookClubGuideA515.pdf.

70. **Sripada C, Angstadt M, Kessler D, Phan KL, Liberzon I, Evans GW,** et al. Volitional regulation of emotions produces distributed alterations in connectivity between visual, attention control, and default networks. Neuroimage. 2014;**89**:110–121.

71. **Caldwell P.** The anger box: Sensory turmoil and pain in autism. Hove, East Sussex, UK: Pavilion Publishing and Media; 2014.

72. **Sterkenburg PS, IJzerman J.** Attachment: A psychotherapeutic treatment. DVD 28 min—includes guidebook. The Netherlands: Bartimeus Reeks; 2007 Available from: https://www.webedu.nl/bestellen/bartimeus/ ?action=order&og=14323, accessed 25 October 2017.

73. **Sterkenburg PS, IJzerman J, de Jong M.** Developing an attachment relationship: Learning together with people with severe multiple disabilities: Part 1. DVD 26 min—includes guidebook. The Netherlands: Bartimeus Reeks; 2010 Available from: https://www.webedu.nl/bestellen/bartimeus/ ?action=order&og=14323.

74. **Sterkenburg PS.** Intervening in stress, attachment and challenging behaviour: Effects in children with multiple disabilities. The Netherlands: Bartimeus Reeks; 2008. Retrieved 2 Aug 2016 from: http://dare. ubvu.vu.nl/bitstream/handle/1871/15813/8494.pdf?sequence=5.

75. **Strain JJ.** Chapter 17: Trauma and stressor-related disorders 2: Adjustment disorders. In: **Leigh H,** Seltzer G, editors. Handbook of consultation-liaison psychiatry. 2nd ed. New York, NY: Springer Science; 2015. p. 243–58.

76. **Keesler JM.** A call for the integration of trauma-informed care among intellectual and developmental disability organizations. J Policy Pract Intellect Disabil. 2014;**11**(1):34–42.

77. **Mevissen L, Lievegoed R, Seubert A, De Jongh A.** Treatment of PTSD in people with severe intellectual disabilities: a case series. Dev Neurorehabil. 2012;**15**(3):223–32.

78. **Emerson E, Einfeld SL.** Challenging behaviour. 3rd ed. Cambridge, UK: Cambridge University Press; 2011.

79. **Bradley E, Caldwell P, Underwood L.** Chapter 16: Autism spectrum disorder. In: Tsakanikos E, McCarthy J, editors. Handbook of psychopathology in intellectual disability: Research, practice, and policy. New York, NY; Heidelberg, Germany: Springer; 2014. p. 237–64.

80. **Wigham S, Hatton C, Taylor JL.** The effects of traumatizing life events on people with intellectual disabilities: a systematic review. J Ment Health Res Intellect Disabil. 2011;4(1):19–39.

81. **Magiati I, Tsakanikos E, Howlin P.** Chapter 9: Psychological and social factors. In: Tsakanikos E, McCarthy JM, editors. Handbook of psychopathology in intellectual disability: Research, practice, and policy. New York: Springer; 2014. p. 123–43.

82. **Pruijssers AC, van Meijel B, Maaskant M, Nijssen W, van Achterberg T.** The relationship between challenging behaviour and anxiety in adults with intellectual disabilities: a literature review. J Intellect Disabil Res. 2014;58(2):162–71.

83. **Helverschou SB, Bakken TL, Martinsen H.** The Psychopathology in Autism Checklist (PAC): a pilot study. Res Autism Spectr Disord. 2009;3(1):179–95.

84. **Hemmings C.** Chapter 4: The relationships between challenging behaviours and psychiatric disorders in people with severe intellectual disabilities. In: **Bouras N,** Holt G, editors. Psychiatric and behavioural disorders in intellectual and developmental disabilities. 2nd ed. Cambridge; New York: Cambridge University Press; 2007. p. 62–75.

85. **Buckles J.** Chapter 3: The epidemiology of psychiatric disorders in adults with intellectual disabilities. In: **Hemmings C,** Bouras N, editors. Psychiatric and behavioral disorders in intellectual and developmental disabilities. 3rd ed. Cambridge, UK: Cambridge University Press; 2016. p. 34–44.

86. **Casey PR.** Chapter 1: Borderline between normal and pathological responses. In: **Casey PR,** Strain JJ, editors. Trauma- and stressor-related disorders: A handbook for clinicians. Arlington,VA: American Psychiatric Association Publishing; 2016. p. 1–22.

87. **Tyrer P.** Chapter 2: Limits to the phenomenological approach to the diagnosis of adjustment disorders. In: **Casey PR,** Strain JJ, editors. Trauma- and stressor-related disorders: A handbook for clinicians. Arlington,VA: American Psychiatric Association Publishing; 2016. p. 23–36.

88. **Slowie D, Ridge K.** The use of medicines in people with learning disabilities. 2015; Retrieved Jul 27, 2016 from: http://www.nhsiq.nhs.uk/media/2671708/keith_ridge_and_dominic_slowie_-_use_of_medicines_in_people_with_learnin....pdf.

Chapter 11

Adjustment disorder: An occupational perspective (with particular focus on the military)

Geoffrey Reid

The diagnostic concept of adjustment disorder (AD), a disturbance of mental state arising specifically as a contingent response to an external psycho-social stressor and relieved on resolution of the stressor, is an apparently simple idea; individuals develop disturbances in mental state in association with psycho-social stressors. However, whilst widely employed as a diagnosis, the evidence base is surprisingly sparse.

AD is a common condition and may impact upon occupational psychiatry either as a direct consequence of the occupation (especially in those occupations exposed to hazardous activities, e.g. the armed forces) or as a result of the associated impairment of AD originating elsewhere impacting upon employability.

AD is associated with both recurrent absence (1) and long-term absence (2), and around 20% never return to work (3). The diagnosis plays an important role in the field of occupational psychiatry, and in particular in the field of military occupational psychiatry, and stress-related disorders are often seen as the particular focus of military psychiatry. AD was the most prevalent mental disorder among UK armed forces personnel in 2015–16, accounting for 35% of all mental disorders in the UK armed forces (4). A study in the Sri Lanka Air Force (5) showed, in a survey of 78 Sri Lankan Air Force personnel referred to psychiatric services, that 25% had a diagnosis of AD, using DSM-IV (*Diagnostic and Statistical Manual of Mental Disorders, Fourth Edition*) criteria. In one UK study (6), the single most commonly diagnosed psychiatric disorder was moderate-to-severe AD in 38.8% of 1,405 personnel seen at a military Department of Community Mental Health (DCMH).

Case vignette 1

Cpl AW was referred to mental health services having been posted from front-line weapons engineering duties on fast jets to weapons instructor duties. He was looking forward to the posting. He had enjoyed his 8 years of Royal Air Force duties and had no previous history of mental health concerns. Although aware that he was never comfortable in front of groups, he had chosen these duties, highly valuing his role as a father and looking for some stability for his family. Unfortunately, he found himself becoming increasingly anxious in the performance of his instructional duties. The posting was for 5 years. His mood deteriorated and he presented to primary care and was referred to the DCMH. At initial CMHN (Community Mental Health Nurse) assessment, he was tearful and low in mood, scoring in the moderately depressed range on the Patient Health Questionnaire (PHQ)-9, and highly anxious. He was avoiding social contact, his affect was flattened, and he was lethargic. His appetite was variably poor but he had not lost weight. He did not have any suicidal thoughts. Antidepressant medication was recommended and commenced in primary care. A consultant psychiatrist review was requested. At consultant review 3 weeks later, he presented as well. He described having developed incapacitating headaches on the medication and he had stopped it after 9 days. The executive had taken action. He had been categorized as unsuited to instructional duties and had been removed from teaching. Action was under way to find him a new posting, returning to his primary weapons engineering task. At further review, he remained well.

The managerial problem-solving was welcome. Medical occupational management would have probably involved a medical recommendation that he was unfit for instructor duties, with an associated medical downgrading. The use of antidepressant medication and the medical downgrading would have precluded a return to front-line weapons engineering duties in the medium term.

Despite being the single most common diagnostic category, there is a remarkable paucity of research into the aetiology and treatment of the disorder, as noted by the various authors of this book. Many community mental health surveys omit AD, and the overall quality of epidemiological studies in either the military or civilian population is poor. The evidence base is not only poor, but almost entirely lacking. Confusion continues to reign in professional and lay circles on the distinction, if any, between depressive and anxiety symptoms arising in association with psycho-social stressors and other forms of anxiety and depressive disorders. Common contemporary treatments seem to focus upon symptom relief, with variable degrees of success, whether by cognitive–behavioural strategies or by medication. Largely, this reflects the current state of psychiatric understanding, where underlying structures and mechanisms remain very incompletely understood.

Unlike much of contemporary medicine, where substantial gains have been made in the understanding of mechanisms, psychiatry remains the last 'clinical art', unsullied by tests and imaging at this point. The attempts to understand and classify psychiatric disorders have been, of necessity, observational and therefore subject to limitations. The use of diagnostic criteria held the hope that discrete categorical disorders would have distinct boundaries, despite the recognition that such boundaries were not reliably determinable for the depressive disorders, resulting in the unitary category of major depression in DSM-III. The situation is neatly summarized by Parker (7): the concept of major depression is analogous to 'major breathlessness'. Breathlessness may arise as a consequence of strong exertion, or disorders such as asthma, emphysema, pneumonia, heart failure, and pulmonary embolus. The classification hides a number of distinct entities, awaiting further knowledge.

Unfortunately, the boundaries within and between diagnostic categories remain fuzzy, and the latest iteration of the DSM classification, DSM-5 (8), remains a symptom-based descriptive system. The inability to clearly identify the nature and mechanisms of psychiatric disorders, how these may operate in 'normality', and the way in which disturbance or decompensation may arise has led to renewed criticism of the validity of psychiatric diagnosis previously seen in the 'anti-psychiatry' days of Thomas Szasz (9). For example, the critique of the DSM operationalization of the diagnosis of depression with inadequate attention to the context has resulted in 'normal sadness' being seen as pathological by Horwitz & Wakefield (10). The deficiencies of symptom-based categorization should be clear: in this, psychiatry remains at the level of physical medicine before the full clarification of physiology, biochemistry, etc. Given these limits in understanding, Spitzer (11) recognized the pragmatic need that expressed disorder needed to be associated with 'clinically significant distress or impairment in social, occupational or other important areas of functioning'. This has remained a feature of the DSM classifications, although it has been weakened in DSM-5 by the statement that 'Mental disorders are *usually* associated with significant distress or disability in social, occupational or other important activities' (italics added) (8). The constraint of functional impairment is central to the practice of military psychiatry.

Military psychiatry is closely integrated with the day-to-day functioning of the armed forces and, as part of a comprehensive military occupational medical service, is required to assess fitness to perform safety-critical tasks and to maintain the workforce. In the UK, mental health care is delivered to the military population from Departments of Community Mental Health, comprising multidisciplinary teams of consultant psychiatrists, clinical psychologists, community mental health nurses (CMHNs), and mental health social workers (MHSWs). The focus on function and fitness for task and the expectation of fitness for task (and the particular safety-critical aspects) have historically been associated with a familiarity with disturbances of mental state arising in association with stressors—most dramatically, of course, in association with operational events, but more mundanely in association with the day-to-day strains of personal and Service life. These circumstances are many and varied. They can include the impact of marital disharmony and family issues, bullying from within the organization, disenchantment with the service, mismatches between individuals and task, separation from families, the growth of single-parent families, and many more aspects of life. A particular issue within the armed forces can be the lack of access to a confidant, arising from the separation of young people from their families. Access to live weapons, the operation of safety-critical equipment, and the high expectation of personnel reliability are intrinsic aspects of the military environment. The identification of disturbances of mental state that arise in association with particular circumstances is critical to the performance of this role in that such identification offers the prospect of ready resolution, whether this is by the process of resolution of stressors or by a specific change in the working environment. Function is the keystone of military occupational psychiatry. For these reasons, adjustment issues have historically played a major role in the day-to-day provision of military mental health services. Military psychiatry was the seedbed for the development of social psychiatry (12) and remains closely embedded with the environmental context of the armed forces.

Disturbances of mental state developing within the operational environment have been widely recognized and have led to a substantial literature on acute stress sisorder (ASD) and post-traumatic stress disorder (PTSD).

ASD has been characterized as an incapacitating disturbance of mental state arising in direct association with operational stressors, and is considered to be commonly transient (80% recovery rate within 72 hours). The symptoms show a typically mixed and changing pattern and can include an initial 'dazed' state, with some constriction of the field of consciousness, and narrowing of attention with an inability to comprehend stimuli and with disorientation. It may be followed by further withdrawal from the surrounding situation (even to the extent of a dissociative stupor) or by agitation and over-reactivity. Although the short-term prognosis is good, it carries an increased risk of PTSD. The disorder is seen as more severe than AD (13).

PTSD is characterized as a long-term chronic disorder with the features of intrusive memories, avoidance, and chronic hyper-arousal. The term post-traumatic stress reaction (PTSR) has been used to identify the development of PTSD-like symptoms in the immediate aftermath of a major stressor, carrying a very high spontaneous recovery rate. PTSR overlaps with the concept of ASD and AD. Most personnel who develop PTSR do not progress to PTSD (14). The NICE (National Institute for Health and Care Excellence) guidelines for PTSD, recognizing the high degree of spontaneous recovery, recommend intervention 3 months after the precipitating event where symptoms persist (15). Within the UK military, the diagnosis of ASD and PTSR within the first 3 months of exposure to a traumatic event is coded as AD, reflecting the use of a computerized, limited diagnostic list. This will inflate the UK military diagnosis of AD, although the major proportion of AD diagnoses are not operationally related.

It has been suggested that AD requires only limited treatment because of a tendency to be short-lived and to resolve spontaneously (16). However, although resolution of symptoms may develop through the process of habituation or by resolution of the precipitating stressor, recovery may be delayed or abolished if the precipitant stressor is maintained or the cognitive appraisal of threat continues. If the stressor persists, the disorder may become persistent (17). However, ICD-10 and DSM-5 require a change of diagnosis where the disorder is persistent, irrespective of the persistence of a precipitating stressor. Such diagnostic practices, whereby the diagnosis may change to major depression where the disorder persists, are a further source of confusion.

A common criticism of the concept of AD is that it is essentially a normal human response to various stressors and therefore not pathological. Horwitz & Wakefield (10), in their critique of 'how psychiatry transformed normal sorrow into depressive disorder', dismiss the concept of AD on the basis that the criterion of impairment of social or occupational functioning fails to exclude large numbers of normal loss response conditions and that virtually any low mood may involve some loss of motivation and interest. They conclude that the flaws in the concept of AD 'are so apparent that researchers and epidemiologists have largely ignored it', the diagnosis suffering from such glaring problems in distinguishing normal from disordered conditions that it has collapsed as a serious target for research under the weight of its own invalidity. Within military psychiatry, function rather than diagnosis remains the prime determinant of occupational intervention and limitations. The determination of fitness to carry out safety-critical tasks is a requirement placed upon military psychiatry. Access to weapons is a common component of military duties, as is the performance of tasks requiring a high level of attention and concentration (e.g. piloting a fast jet), and the presence of any self-harmful thoughts or the extent of actual and anticipated impairment of concentration and attention is an essential component of military psychiatric assessment. The specific diagnosis is a secondary issue.

Case vignette 2

LCpl AB, a Royal Signals operator, was referred after having presented with poor sleep, distress, and low mood. His girlfriend had been raped. She had developed PTSD, for which she was receiving treatment. He described taking hours to get to sleep, being subject to ruminative thoughts. His appetite was good, and his libido variable. Concentration was variable. He did not understand what was happening to his girlfriend. At CMHN assessment, he scored within the moderately severely depressed range on the PHQ-9. A high-achiever at school, he had been the victim of bullying and had been expelled from school for poor behaviour but had enjoyed his army career. He had no previous psychiatric history. He had served for 4 years; he had not been on any operational deployments. He did not have routine access to weapons and he was not involved in safety-critical activities. He did not have any self-harmful thoughts or wish to be dead. He was not considered to require any medical functional limitations. CMHN management included psycho-education on PTSD and the introduction of coping strategies for ruminative thoughts. He settled, his mood improved, and the ruminative thoughts receded. He remained well at follow up.

Development of the concept

The concept of AD is closely related to wider concepts of stress and has deep historical roots.

An early understanding derives from the work of Yerkes & Dodson (18) in 1908, describing the relationship between arousal and performance: the human performance curve (or 'Yerkes–Dodson curve'). As arousal increases, performance (both physical and mental) increases. However, when arousal becomes too high, performance is impaired. Different tasks require different levels of arousal for optimum performance, with difficult cognitive tasks requiring lower levels of arousal than those demanding stamina or persistence. Diamond et al. (19) showed that there was a relationship with circulating levels of stress hormones which showed an inverted-U relationship with memory performance.

The original Yerkes–Dodson curve is shown below (see Fig. 11.1).

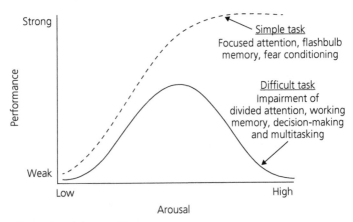

Fig. 11.1 The Yerkes–Dodson curve.
Reproduced from Journal of Comparative Neurology and Psychology, 18(5), Yerkes RM, Dodson JD, The relation of strength of stimulus to rapidity of habit-formation, pp. 459–482, Copyright 1908, with permission from The Wistar Institute of Anatomy and Biology.

During the World War I, the symptoms of shell shock and flying stress were identified in terms of the fear and fatigue associated with prolonged exposure to operational environments. The concepts of stability of the internal environment deriving from Claude Bernard in the nineteenth century, and the work of Walter Cannon (20) and others during the 1920s and 1930s, in turn led to the concept of the preservation of homeostasis. From 1936 onwards, and predominantly after the World War II, Hans Selye (21, 22) was responsible for developing his concept of the general adaptation syndrome and the understanding of the activity of the hypothalamic-pituitary-adrenal axis. The discovery that rats responded to various forms of damaging stimuli with a general response that involved alarm, resistance, and exhaustion led to the formulation of the general adaptation syndrome, which was said to consist of the following three stages: an initial alarm or shock phase, a stage of adaptation to injury in which physiological resistance allowed normal function, and a final stage of exhaustion when adaptive mechanism failed.

The role of stressors in the development of illness was pursued. Holmes & Rahe (23) developed the Social Adjustment Rating Scale, attempting to quantify stressful life events such as bereavement, divorce, and illness and to provide a means of predicting the development of illness. In 1970, Rahe tested the validity of the scale in a study of 2,500 US sailors. They were asked to rate scores of 'life events' over the previous 6 months. Over the next 6 months, detailed records were kept of the sailors' health. There was a +0.118 correlation between stress scale scores and illness. In 1978, Brown & Harris (24) identified three factors that affected the development of depressive mood in women: protective factors, vulnerability factors, and provoking agents in women. Protective factors (e.g. high levels of intimacy with one's husband) were found to protect against development of depression in spite of stressors. These factors lead to higher levels of self-esteem and the possibility of finding other sources of meaning in life. Vulnerability factors were found to increase the risk of depression in combination with particularly stressful life events— called 'provoking agents' in the study. The most significant vulnerability factors were:

1. Loss of one's mother before the age of 11
2. Lack of a confiding relationship

3. More than three children under the age of 14 at home

4. Unemployment. Provoking agents were found to contribute to acute and ongoing stress.

These stressors could result in grief and hopelessness in vulnerable women with no social support. In 1988, Bebbington et al. (25), in the Camberwell Collaborative Depression Study, showed that the onset of depressive symptoms was associated with life stressors; the hypothesis that the 'endogenous' group of disorders would be relatively independent of prior life stress was not confirmed. Mazure (26) summarized the findings, noting that stressors were 2.5 times more likely in depressed patients than in controls, and that in community samples 80% of depressed cases had preceding major life events, and Hammen (27) noted that there was an established, robust, and causal association between stressful life events and major depressive episodes.

Stress has now long been identified as a risk factor for major depressive disorder, and a large body of evidence is implicating a dysregulated endocrine and inflammatory response system in its pathogenesis. Hughes et al. (28) provide a review of the role of the immune system and stressors in the onset of major depression. The desire to be free of the aetiological considerations inherent in the older concepts of reactive or neurotic depression and endogenous depression concept led to the use of the term 'major depression' and a general perception that depression was a unitary phenomenon. However, Goldberg (29) reiterated that major depression is not a homogeneous entity. He noted that depression could arise as a toxic reaction to drugs or could result from endocrine disorders such as myxoedema or Cushing's syndrome, and that the depressed phase of bi-polar illness could be indistinguishable from unipolar depression. He discussed five subtypes and notes that many milder cases of depression remit without specific treatment, suggesting that they are 'homeostatic responses to stress'. The biological mechanisms remain unclear, but it is this variety that is encompassed in the category of depressive adjustment disorder. Evidence is beginning to emerge on the differences between AD and major depression. Lindqvist et al. (30) showed that in individuals with suicidal ideation, post-dexamethasone suppression of cortisol levels was negatively correlated with symptom scores only in those with a clinical diagnosis of major depression. There was no correlation in those diagnosed with AD. Individuals developing AD in the context of workplace bullying did not develop abnormal dexamethasone suppression test results (31). For further information on the psychobiology of AD, see Chapter 5.

Occupational stressors

In the occupational field, the armed forces environment is characterized not only by the risk of exposure to the challenging circumstances of operational deployments, but also by a disciplined, structured environment in which individuals surrender some of their abilities to make environmental choices. Moreover, the services are also characterized by stoical attitudes, forged in the heat of operational demands, whereby intolerance of physical and mental hardship is discouraged, both by training and custom (32). Within this environment, the possibility of changes in circumstances, either geographically or socially, is surrounded by constraints and limitations. Individuals cannot easily remove themselves from an environment or make changes in their social milieu. Young people, removed from the buffering effects of social support in their home environment, may not find alternative sources of confiding support readily available. The capacity to resolve stressful circumstances may be constrained.

In operational deployments, armed forces personnel may be overwhelmed by the intrinsic challenges or develop stress reactions that may be best categorized as AD, prompting psychiatric aeromedical evacuation. AD is a common cause of psychiatric aeromedical evacuation. These post-trauma stress reactions have a high spontaneous recovery rate; the diagnostic category of PTSD would not generally be applied until 3 months after the incident, although this does not preclude early treatment.

It has been suggested that the great advantage of occupational psychiatry in the armed forces is the ability to make changes to the working environment. In the day-to-day working situation, where local environmental problems are not resolvable and it is judged that re-location of the individual is likely to result in a sustained improvement (e.g. in cases of personality clashes, bullying), there is the possibility of a geographical move. In the UK armed forces there are restricted opportunities for such moves within the organization of the Royal Navy and the Army, but more opportunities within the Royal Air Force, reflecting its more homogeneous corporate structure. This is recognized in the specific provision of a psychiatric recommendation for a geographical posting to enable effective psychiatric management. This would be for a maximum of 12 months and carries a requirement for a return to full effectiveness.

Controversy has arisen in the USA with the discharge of personnel from the military with a diagnosis of AD, with allegations of it being used to get rid of 'troublemakers, whistle-blowers, sexual assault complainants, and ill or injured service members'. In many cases this reflects disaffection and demotivation with the military working environment—a mismatch between the individual and the conditions of the military environment, a stressor resulting in the appearance of adjustment features—rather than formal psychiatric disorder arising from operational experiences. In the UK, policies to address this issue remain from the days of conscription. These were developed prior to the inclusion of AD in the classification systems and are couched in terms of 'temperamental unsuitability'. Each service has its own Temperamental Unsuitability Policy, with no identified common ground other than the need to expedite the discharge of a disaffected individual. Although a managerial and not a medical discharge, each policy requires individuals to be seen by a psychiatrist who then recommends discharge under the relevant policy. The Royal Navy requires the psychiatrist to classify the sailor according to a system of establishing the severity of personality traits and the potential for intervention. The Army requires the psychiatrist to state that the individual is 'temperamentally unsuitable'. Finally, the Royal Air Force requires the psychiatrist to certificate that the individual is not suffering from any remedial psychiatric disorder. These policies may be seen as historical artefacts, serving to facilitate the discharge of those who no longer wish to serve in the military. The prospects for approaching these policies in terms of AD with poor prognosis in the military setting are probably unlikely.

Management

Outside the military environment, while AD is widely recognized as highly prevalent, there remains remarkably little research on the course, outcomes, or treatment. Guidelines have been developed in the Netherlands (3) recommending treatment based on cognitive–behavioural principles, predominantly stress inoculation training and graded activity, aiming to enhance problem-solving capacity.

Historically, management of AD in the workplace has focused pragmatically on a combination of problem-solving and stress management techniques. A meta-analysis (33) of relaxation training (Jacobson's progressive relaxation, autogenic training, applied relaxation, and meditation) has shown consistent and significant efficacy in reducing anxiety. The Cochrane Database (34) has published a meta-analysis, finding moderate-quality evidence that cognitive–behavioural therapy did not significantly reduce time until partial return to work, and low-quality evidence that it did not significantly reduce time to full return to work, compared with no treatment. Moderate-quality evidence showed that problem-solving therapy significantly enhanced partial return to work at 1-year follow up compared to non-guideline-based care, but did not significantly enhance time to full return to work at 1-year follow up. An important limitation was the small number of studies included in the meta-analyses and the small number of participants, which lowered the power of the analyses.

The configuration of UK military psychiatry into 15 Departments of Community Mental Health, facilitating local access, and the delivery of front-line psychiatric care by uniformed community mental health nurses, encourages the acquisition of familiarity with the military environment and the development of knowledge of the availability of problem-solving solutions (35) within the structured military environment.

Symptomatic treatment of anxiety and insomnia with benzodiazepines and hypnotics is often used, but in 1988 the Committee on Safety of Medicines (36) responded to the widespread misuse of benzodiazepines and concerns over the development of pharmacological dependence by issuing guidelines that they should be used for short-term use for 2–4 weeks only. The guidelines were reinforced in 2012 (37). Antidepressant medication may have benefits by virtue of sedative and anxiolytic properties. Such drugs may also have a direct effect on reducing ruminative thought. There has been no published evidence on which antidepressant drugs might be most helpful in treating AD, but a protocol for a Cochrane systematic review of pharmacological interventions in AD in adults has been published and the work is ongoing (38).

Patients with a clinical diagnosis of AD are likely to overlap with individuals seen by other agencies, including social work. Task-centred casework is a well-established treatment model in social work (39).

A systematic review (40) of the quantitative and qualitative literature on workplace-based return-to-work interventions, albeit not addressed to AD but limited to patients with pain-related conditions, recommended that workplace-based return-to-work interventions included the following core disability management strategies: early s upportive contact with the worker, the offer of work accommodation, and contact between the healthcare provider and the workplace. There was moderate evidence that interventions which include these three components lead to important reductions in work disability duration and in associated costs. There is mixed evidence that these programmes lead to improvements in quality-of-life outcomes. Such conditions are met by effective occupational health departments and personnel. This model could potentially be applied to and tested in those with AD in occupational settings.

Occupational prognosis

In a study (41) of 328 young military conscripts with a DSM-IV diagnosis of AD secondary to non-combat military stress, the diagnosis was closely associated with undisturbed psycho-social function outside military life. A further study (42) of over 2,000 US naval personnel found that AD was less severe and less disabling than other psychiatric conditions, being shorter and with higher levels of subsequent return to effective work. In the Sri Lankan study (2), four-fifths returned to work within 6 months.

Individuals may be able to continue at work, with restrictions in place reflecting their capacity to work and the need for safety. The armed forces have a comprehensive fitness-for-work medical grading system that allows workplace restrictions to be put in place by the medical services without communicating confidential medical information. It is preferable to retain an individual in work where possible, albeit in a restricted role, thereby minimizing the hurdles of a return to work. However, where an individual is unable to work, sickness absence may become inevitable, though effective management is likely to reduce the period away from work.

Developments in classification

The establishment of a working group for disorders specifically associated with stress for ICD-11 has resulted in the proposed cluster under a single category of 'Disorders Specifically Associated with Stress'. These comprise post-traumatic stress disorder, complex post-traumatic stress disorder, adjustment disorder, and prolonged grief disorder (43).

The symptom pattern for AD is characterized by 'preoccupation with the stressor and failure to adapt'. Subtypes of AD have not been shown to have any clinical utility and have been abandoned. Acute stress reaction is not included, being moved to 'Conditions Associated with Psychosocial Circumstances' because of perceptions of ambiguity of definition and its transient time course. Until ICD-11 is published, the ICD-10 definition remains in place. It is unclear whether the new definition of AD will identify the same group as do the current criteria. This is particularly important in the context of defence forces, where the symptom overlap between the proposed ICD-11 criteria for AD (preoccupation and avoidance are among the core and secondary symptoms, respectively) and PTSD may cause diagnostic confusion. Alternatively, AD may be seen as a subthreshold form of PTSD. The defence forces will be a crucial population in which to clarify the utility and validity of the proposed new criteria.

Summary

The diagnosis of AD forms a substantial proportion of the clinical diagnoses in the field of armed forces occupational psychiatry. To a large degree, this is likely to reflect the functional orientation of military psychiatry, where the impact on performance and safety-critical tasks has a high priority. The concept has developed against the background of almost a century's work on the role of stressors on mental states. While it is now generally accepted that a robust relationship exists between the development of major depression and stressors, it is being recognized that major depression is not a homogeneous entity and that there is a variety of depressive disorders that may remit without specific treatment. Evidence is beginning to develop of biological differences between major depression and depressive adjustment disorder. Problem-solving and stress management strategies are the current main ingredients of the management of AD, and the condition carries a good prognosis for a return to work, but there is a paucity of treatment and outcome studies. Developments in classification are to be incorporated in ICD-11, which may help to operationalize the diagnosis.

References

1. Koopmans PC, Bültmann U, Roelen CAM, Hoedeman R, van der Klink JJ, Groothoff JW. Recurrence of sickness absence due to common mental disorders. Int Arch Occup Environ Health. 2011;**84**(2):193–201.

2. Catalina-Romero C, Pastrana-Jiménez JI, Tenas-López MJ, Martínez-Muñoz P, Ruiz-Moraga M, Fernández-Labandera C, et al. Long-term sickness absence due to adjustment disorder. Occup Med (Lond). 2012;**62**(5):375–8.

3. van der Klink KJ, van den Dijk FJ. Dutch practice guidelines for managing adjustment disorders in occupational and primary health care. Scand J Work Environ Health. 2003;**29**(6):478–87.

4. UK Armed Forces Mental Health Annual Summary & Trend Over Time, 2007/8–2015/16, UK Ministry of Defence, Jun 16.

5. Perera H, Suveedran T, Mariestella A. Profile of psychiatric disorders in the Sri Lanka Air Force and the outcome at 6 months. Mil Med. 2004;**169**:396–9.

6. Jones N. The long term occupational fitness of UK military personnel following community mental health care. J Ment Health. 2017 Jun **24**:1–8. doi: 10.1080/09638237.2017.1340596 [Epub ahead of print]

7. Parker G. A case for reprising and redefining melancholia. Can J Psychiatry. 2013;**58**:183–9.

8. American Psychiatric Association. Diagnostic and statistical manual of mental disorders. 5th ed. Arlington, VA: American Psychiatric Association; 2013.

9. Szasz TS. The myth of mental illness. New York: Hoeber-Harper; 1961.

10. Horwitz AV, Wakefield JC. The loss of sadness. New York: Oxford University Press; 2007.

11. Spritzer R. The diagnostic status of homosexuality in SM-III: a reformulation of the issues. Am J Psychiatry. 1981;**138**(2):210–15.

12. Leff J. The historical development of social psychiatry. In: Morgan C, Bhugra D, editors. Principles of social psychiatry. 2nd ed. Wiley-Blackwell; 2010.

13. **Reid GE.** Aviation psychiatry. In: Ernsting's aviation and space medicine. 5th ed. CRC Press; 2016.

14. **Harrison J, Sharpley J, Greenberg N.** The management of post traumatic reactions in the military. J R Army Med Corps. 2008;**154**(2):110–14.

15. **NICE (National Institute for Health and Care Excellence).** Post-traumatic stress disorder: Management. Clinical guideline CG26, 2005.

16. **Strain JJ, Diefenbacher A.** The adjustment disorders: the conundrums of the diagnoses. Compr Psychiatry. 2008;**49**(2):121–30.

17. **Andreasen N, Hoenk P.** The predictive value of adjustment disorders: a follow-up study. Am J Psychiatry. 1982;**139**:584–90.

18. **Yerkes RM, Dodson JD.** The relation of strength of stimulus to rapidity of habit-formation. J Comp Neurol Psychol. 1908;**18**(5):459–82.

19. **Diamond DM, Campbell AM, Park CR, Halonen J, Zoladz PR.** The temporal dynamics model of emotional memory processing: a synthesis on the neurobiological basis of stress-induced amnesia, flashbulb and traumatic memories, and the Yerkes-Dodson law. Neural Plast. 2007;**2007**:60803.

20. **Cannon WB.** The wisdom of the body. New York: WW Norton; 1932.

21. **Selye H.** A syndrome produced by diverse nocuous agents. Nature. 1936;**138**:32.

22. **Selye H.** Stress and the general adaptation syndrome. Br Med J. 1950;**1**(4667):1383–92.

23. **Holmes TH, Rahe RH.** The Social Readjustment Rating Scale. J Psychosom Res. 1967;**11**(2):213–18.

24. **Brown GW, Harris TO.** Social origins of depression: A study of psychiatric disorder in women. London: Tavistock; 1978.

25. **Bebbington P, Brugha T, MacCarthy B, Potter J, Sturt E, Wykes T, et al.** The Camberwell Collaborative Depression Study. I. Depressed probands: adversity and the form of depression. Br J Psychiatry. 1988;**152**:754–65.

26. **Mazure CM.** Life stressors as risk factors in depression. Clin Psychol Sci Pract. 1998;**5**:291–313.

27. **Hammen C.** Stress and depression. Annu Rev Clin Psychol. 2005;**1**:293–319.

28. **Hughes MM, Connor TJ, Harkin A.** Stress-related immune markers in depression: implications for treatment. Int J Neuropsychopharmacol. 2016;**19**(6):pyw001.

29. **Goldberg D.** The heterogeneity of 'major depression'. World Psychiatry. 2011;**10**(3):226–8.

30. **Lindqvist D, Träskman-Bendz L, Vang, F.** Suicidal intent and the HPA-axis characteristics of suicide attempters with major depression and adjustment disorders. Arch Suicide Res. 2008;**12**:197–207.

31. **Rocco A, Martocchia A, Frugoni P, Baldini R, Sani G, Di Simone Di Giuseppe B, et al.** Inverse correlation between morning cortisol levels and MMPI psychasthenia and depression scale scores in victims of mobbing with adjustment disorders. Neuro Endocrinol Lett. 2007;**28**:610–13.

32. **Sherman N.** Stoic warriors: The ancient philosophy behind the military mind. USA: Oxford University Press; 2005.

33. **Manzoni GM, Pagnini F, Castelnuovo G, Molinari E.** Relaxation training for anxiety: a ten-years systematic review with meta-analysis, BMC Psychiatry. 2008;**8**:41.

34. **Arends I, Bruinvels DJ, Rebergen DS, Nieuwenhuijsen K, Madan I, Neumeyer-Gromen A,** et al. Interventions to facilitate return to work in adults with adjustment disorders. Cochrane Database Syst Rev. 2012;**12**: CD006389.

35. **Hawton K, Salkovskis PM, Kirk J, Clark DM.** Problem-solving. In: Cognitive behaviour therapy for psychiatric problems. Hawton K, editor. USA: Oxford University Press; 1989.

36. **Committee on Safety of Medicines (CSM).** Benzodiazepines, dependence and withdrawal symptoms. UK government bulletin to prescribing doctors. Current Problems. 1988; number 21:1–2.

37. **Mehdi T.** Benzodiazepines revisited. Br J Med Pract. 2012;**5**(1):a501.

38. **Casey P, Pillay D, Wilson L, Maercker A, Rice A, Kelly B.** Pharmacological interventions for adjustment disorders in adults (Protocol). Cochrane Database Syst Rev. 2013; Issue 6. Art. No.: CD010530. DOI: 10.1002/14651858

39. **Reid WJ, Epstein L.** Task-centred casework. New York: Columbia University Press; 1972.

40. **Franche, R-L.** Institute for Work & Health, 2004

41. **Bonelli RM, Bugram R.** Additional A-criterion for adjustment disorders? Can J Psychiatry. 2000;**45**(8):763.

42. **Looney J, Gunderson E.** Transient situational disturbances course and outcome. Am J Psychiatry. 1978;**135**:660–3.

43. **Maercker A, Brewin CR, Bryant RA, Cloitre M, Reed GM, van Ommeren M,** et al. Proposals for mental disorders specifically associated with stress in the International Classification of Diseases-11. Lancet. 2013;**381**(9878):1683–5.

Chapter 12

Adjustment disorders in legal settings

Keith Rix

COUNSEL: Dr White, you have made a diagnosis of adjustment disorder. What specific criteria have you have applied?

DOCTOR: I have made my diagnosis on the basis of clinical judgement.

COUNSEL: I am sure that you have applied your clinical judgement, as no doubt Dr Black has done, but she has not made a diagnosis of adjustment disorder. Please answer my question: What are the specific criteria you have applied?

COUNSEL: Dr Brown, you have made a diagnosis of adjustment disorder. There is no dispute that, for about 6 weeks following the accident, Mr Smith was distressed, he required 4 days off work, he was occasionally distracted at work by thoughts of the accident, although no one at work noticed or commented, except a close friend, and about one night a week he had trouble getting to sleep thinking about the accident and worrying about another one. Your colleague Dr Green says that this is a normal response to an accident of the sort that Mr Smith had. Surely distress, anxiety, low mood, and so on are universal features of the human condition in certain circumstances? Why do you call it an adjustment disorder?

COUNSEL: Dr Lamb, you have made a diagnosis of adjustment disorder. The court has heard from Dr Wolf that, although you agree about the symptoms Mrs Jones has suffered, she does not accept that they amount to a mental disorder as such; she would not say that Mrs Jones has a recognized medical condition. You have agreed with her that her symptoms are not sufficient to make a diagnosis of even a mild depressive episode and her evidence is that you psychiatrists use the term 'adjustment disorder' for what you call subthreshold conditions that are mild and do not meet the criteria for another mental disorder. So, we have here a milder-than-mild state of depression which you agree does not cross the threshold for making a diagnosis of any recognized mental disorder. There is no dispute about Mrs Jones being very unhappy that her father was suffering so much with terminal cancer, but are you telling the court that this state of unhappiness, or depression as you want to call it, was so different from the experience any other loving daughter would have had in those circumstances that it reflected a recognized medical condition and caused such a substantial impairment of her ability to form a rational judgement and exercise self-control that it explains her smothering and killing her father with a pillow?

COUNSEL: Dr Hawke, you have ruled out the diagnosis of adjustment disorder because there is no evidence of significant impairment of functioning and in doing so you rely on what is called ICD-11. Dr Dove says that according to the American DSM-5, which is also widely used outside of the USA, functional impairment is not necessary for a diagnosis of adjustment disorder and, according to ICD-10, although interference with social functioning and performance is usual in an adjustment disorder, it is not necessary for the diagnosis. Furthermore, Dr Dove points out that the ICD-11 criteria to which you refer are criteria for research. Please tell the court about the evidence which justifies the ICD-11 criterion that there must be significant impairment of everyday functioning.

These four hypothetical examples illustrate some of the potential pitfalls for the expert psychiatric witness that can arise from three controversial aspects of adjustment disorders identified by Strain & Casey (2016): (1) the absence of specific criteria resulting in a reliance or over-reliance on clinical judgement, (2) the distinction between normal and abnormal responses to stress, (3) their status as subthreshold disorders. The fourth is illustrative of the potential difficulty resulting from the difference between ICD-11 and DSM-5 in terms of the requirement of significant functional impairment and the risks of relying on ICD diagnostic criteria for research rather than on clinical descriptions and diagnostic guidelines. As happened in the case of *R (on the application of B) v Dr SS, Responsible Medical Officer and Others* (1), the courts may be unwilling to accept reliance on diagnostic criteria for research and prefer instead to rely on those criteria applicable to the clinical setting.

This chapter is in two parts. The first part examines the approaches taken by courts in cases where adjustment disorders have featured. In the second part, the lessons that can be learned from these cases are translated into guidance for expert witnesses in cases where a diagnosis of adjustment disorder (AD) is made or is at issue.

The legal landscape

The civil jurisdiction

In industrialized nations, the civil cases in which psychiatrists are most likely to be instructed are personal injury cases brought following road traffic and industrial accidents and actions for alleged medical negligence where psychiatric evidence may be sought as to the psychiatric consequences of the allegedly negligent treatment.

In England and Wales, personal injuries are 'any disease and any impairment of a person's physical or mental condition' (s 38, Limitation Act 1980). Although there are controversies concerning the nature of adjustment disorders, these have figured little in personal injury litigation. The courts accept adjustment disorders as types of psychiatric injury and award compensation according to the Judicial College guidelines (2), which set out the following categories of damage: 'less severe', 'moderate', 'moderately severe', and 'severe'.

The courts can also award damages for 'nervous shock'—pure psychiatric injury unaccompanied by any physical injury, as for example suffered by a road traffic accident victim who is physically unharmed but witnesses, and reacts to, the horrendous injuries of the victims (3). Here, the law is very clear that damages will be awarded only for 'a recognizable psychiatric illness' (4) and not, for example, 'for the emotional distress which any normal person experiences when someone he loves is killed or injured' (5). There is no case law here involving adjustment disorders, but this is clearly a circumstance in which it might be argued that the symptoms of the AD were symptoms that did not amount to a recognizable psychiatric illness.

By contrast, there are a number of circumstances involving torts of trespass to the person and harassment and breach of contract in which compensation may be awarded for what has been termed 'mere mental or emotional distress' (6). Examples include anger and indignation at unnecessary dental treatment, hurt feelings after wrongful eviction, distress on having one's photographs used in advertisements for pornographic magazines, injury to peace of mind caused by the imminent collapse of a house, or a disappointing holiday, and distress on being sold a faulty car (7). In such cases it might not matter if the person's reaction is so normal that a diagnosis of AD cannot be made, but if it is, such a diagnosis should be more than sufficient to establish a cause of action.

Courting controversy

The case of *Dodd v Wright* (8) illustrates how close the courts have come to the controversial nature of AD. The claimant had a psychiatric report with the diagnosis of AD. A district judge ruled that there was no evidence to persuade the court to consider that there was a psychiatric disorder and ruled that she was unable to rely on the report. On appeal, the court found that:

> "if by those words the judge was indicating that the claimant did not suffer from a recognised psychiatric illness, it may be that he was correct. There could have been a technical debate whether adjustment disorder, as opposed to recognised psychiatric injury such as post-traumatic stress disorder and depression, amounts to a psychiatric illness as such".

Normal or abnormal?

The case of *McCarroll v Northern Ireland Housing Executive* (9) typifies the case in which the argument is whether the person's experience is normal or abnormal. The issue was whether the plaintiff suffered from a psychiatric condition as a result of stress at work. One psychiatrist considered that she was suffering from an AD. The other psychiatrist felt that she was simply suffering upset and feelings of anger and frustration as the result of her work problems. In choosing to favour the assessment made by the former, the court noted that a specialist in occupational health who carried out an assessment on the plaintiff at the request of the defendant had concluded that the plaintiff developed 'a significant adjustment reaction to the situation in work in which she perceives herself to be a victim of harassment and subsequently unfair treatment', so the court found that in the wake of the disciplinary process the plaintiff was suffering from a work-related adjustment disorder.

In *Webb v Norfolk & Norwich University Hospital NHS Trust* (10), a case of unsatisfactory breast reconstruction, the court rode roughshod over the distinction between what was regarded by one expert as understandable distress and anger, and in which no formal diagnosis was founded, and what the other diagnosed as an adjustment disorder:

> I take into account ... the psychiatric consequences described by the psychiatrists in this case, who are essentially agreed that, although the claimant is not suffering from clinical depression as such, she has what Dr X described as an adjustment disorder, and although Dr Y makes no formal diagnosis to that effect, they are effectively talking about the same thing, and he describes distress and anger on the part of the claimant.

In the case of *Tarakhil v The Home Office* (11) damages were awarded for false imprisonment and wrongful detention and for the psychiatric consequences of that detention. The claimant had been clearly deeply shocked by his initial detention, with symptoms of anxiety and fear of both detention and deportation, and he had displayed clear signs of AD with anxiety features. He was awarded damages in the 'less severe' category.

In the case of *Manzi v King's College Hospital NHS Foundation Trust* (12) the experts agreed that, but for the problems with the retained products of conception, the claimant would not have suffered from an AD. They disagreed as to the length of time it had lasted, but the parties were agreed that the Judicial Studies Board's Guidelines'[1] 'moderate' bracket for psychiatric harm gave the appropriate range. However, the psychiatrists disagreed as to whether the claimant had suffered a second period of AD during her pregnancy with her third child. In her statement the claimant said that she had become very anxious

---

[1] Now published by the Judicial College—see reference 2

and scared when she was pregnant with her third child. She said that all of the emotions that she had experienced following the previous birth came flooding back, and that caused her a lot of distress. One psychiatrist recognized that her fear was that there would be similar complications after this third delivery, but he did not consider that her condition during this pregnancy was sufficient to constitute a mental illness. In their joint report the experts' difference of view was repeated, with Dr X maintaining that there had been no second period of mental illness, and with Dr Y saying that there had been and that it had lasted for about 8 months. The court accepted that the events following the earlier birth had been traumatic for the claimant and, as asserted by Dr Y, accepted that this had led to a recurrence of AD, not merely the subclinical [sic] symptoms, as Dr X had described. It was estimated that this had lasted no less than 6 months and would therefore attract a further award towards the bottom of the 'moderate' bracket.

It is interesting that although the condition of AD could in itself have been regarded as a subclinical condition, in this case it was symptoms not amounting to an adjustment disorder that were regarded as subclinical.

'Psychiatric damage generally' or 'post-traumatic stress disorder'

It is worth noting that the Judicial College guidelines separate 'psychiatric damage generally' from 'post-traumatic stress disorder'. However, they include under 'psychiatric damage generally' cases in which there is 'an element of compensation for post-traumatic stress disorder' and state that where it does figure, any award will be towards the upper end of the bracket. With the exception of the 'severe' category, awards for cases categorized under 'post-traumatic stress disorder' (PTSD) are all considerably higher than for psychiatric damage generally. This would explain the anecdotal experience of some experts who have been under pressure to diagnose PTSD rather than adjustment disorder. Insofar as the proposed ICD-11 research diagnostic criteria embody a concept of AD that may not be sufficiently distinct from PTSD, with symptom descriptions that emphasize the similarity of the two disorders (Bachem & Casey (13)), this may become a more fraught and contentious area given that the 'label' seems to have implications for the level of compensation.

The criminal jurisdiction

Although there are a number of defences in connection with which psychiatric evidence may be admissible, there are probably only two defences in relation to which evidence of AD is likely to be admissible. They are the partial defence of diminished responsibility to a charge of murder and the partial defence (hereinafter 'defence') of infanticide. It is highly unlikely that a diagnosis of AD could form the basis of a defence of insanity as there is nothing in its psychopathology that would account for the defect of reasoning which the *M'Naghten Rule* would require to be satisfied. Equally unlikely is it that such a diagnosis could be the basis for arguing that a defendant did not have the *mens rea* or intention to commit the crime, as the following two cases illustrate.

Adjustment disorder irrelevant

An unsuccessful attempt to use evidence of AD to overturn a conviction for fraud is illustrated by the case of *R v Hayes* (14). It reveals the need to show how the psychopathology may explain the person's behaviour. The appellant had been convicted of conspiracy to manipulate the Japanese yen LIBOR (London Interbank Offered Rate). It was a ground for appeal that the trial judge had been wrong to rule inadmissible evidence of the appellant's mental ill-health, specifically an AD (mixed anxiety and depressive reaction). It was argued that this evidence was relevant to his state of mind and understanding when he entered into a formal agreement in which he admitted that he had acted dishonestly. The Court of Appeal rejected this. It accepted the trial judge's finding that there was no evidence that the appellant did not understand the process into which he entered or that his depressed emotional state impacted on his comprehension; indeed, there was nothing in the medical evidence to support such an assertion. It accepted the trial judge's finding that the appellant himself had never suggested that his mental state had impacted on the conclusion of the agreement or his ability to understand it or to make a rational decision about entering into the agreement. The Court of Appeal added that the jury did not need medical evidence to understand the pressure (and consequent distress) that the appellant must have endured. In this case the expert had not expressed the opinion that the AD had affected the appellant's state of mind at the time he entered into the agreement, but the appellant's counsel, on appeal, wanted to persuade the court that the AD had indeed affected the appellant.

Another unsuccessful reliance on the diagnosis of AD is illustrated by the case of *R v Moffat* (15). This was a court martial case, and the seaman was convicted of using a firearm with intent to cause another to believe that unlawful violence would be used. There was psychiatric evidence that he was suffering at the time from an AD which so affected his emotions and behaviour that his judgement was impaired. As a result, he acted completely out of character. The disorder was temporary, brought about by his ruminating on his earlier failure to be present to support his wife while she was in a difficult labour. The court found that it did not provide any defence, and accordingly there was not much to distinguish this seaman from many others who instantly regret their decisions. However, the court accepted and emphasized its acceptance that the appellant acted out of character.

Diminished responsibility

When my former colleague Dr John Kent was teaching trainee psychiatrists about diminished responsibility, he showed a list of psychiatric disorders which had been accepted as the basis for the defence and a list of those which had not been accepted. The two lists were identical and they included adjustment disorders. At that time the partial defence in England and Wales had not undergone the reform brought about by section 52 of the Criminal Justice Act 2009. It is probably now even less likely that an adjustment disorder will successfully found the defence.

The defence has four ingredients: (1) abnormality of mental functioning; (2) a recognized medical condition from which it arises; (3) substantial impairment of the mental responsibility to do any one of three defined things—(a) to understand their own conduct, (b) to form a rational judgment, and (c) to exercise self-control; and (4) an explanation for the killing being provided by the abnormality of mental functioning. There are a number of significant hurdles here if the diagnosis is one of AD.

The test for abnormality of mental functioning is likely to continue to be the 'abnormality of mind' test set out in the case of *R v Byrne* (16): 'a state of mind so different from that of ordinary human beings that the reasonable man would term it abnormal'. But the state of mind of someone with an AD is not very different at all from that of an ordinary person under some particular stress. A leading Scottish authority (*HM Advocate v Savage* (17) on diminished responsibility refers to 'a state of mind … bordering on, although not amounting to, insanity'. The state of mind of someone with an AD is a long way from the border of insanity. The allocation of adjustment disorders to a subthreshold category of mental disorders is evidence that psychiatrists regard the state of mind as not so different from that of ordinary human beings under stress. If experts on mental states do not regard adjustment disorders as sufficiently abnormal to cross the threshold and amount to actual mental disorders, lay jurors are probably even less likely to regard them as reflecting a state of mind so different from ordinary human beings under stress that they would term it abnormal.

Similar points can be made about the concept of 'a recognized medical condition'. Here, 'recognized' does not mean recognized by doctors; it means recognized by the courts. Given the subthreshold status of adjustment disorders it would not be surprising to find a judge ruling against their recognition as actual medical conditions. So far that has not happened, and in at least three cases the court has accepted that an AD is a recognized medical condition.

In the case of *R v Webb* (18), where the defendant killed his sick wife who believed, without medical evidence, that her cancer had recurred, AD was accepted as being a recognized medical condition. Two psychiatrists gave expert evidence about the practical effect of the defendant's adjustment disorder:

> As it developed, it became increasingly difficult for him to make even simple domestic decisions and simple telephone calls. The disorder was described as a state of subjective distress and emotional disturbance which interfered with social functioning and performance.

The psychiatric evidence was that towards the end of her life the appellant would have found it difficult to resist the pressure from his wife to step in, if it became necessary, to finish her life for her. That is what she wanted. That is what she said on many occasions. When the Court of Appeal considered the appellant's appeal against the sentence of 2 years' imprisonment that had been imposed, it observed that the psychiatric evidence accorded with the jury's verdict 'that at the very least the appellant was suffering from a significant adjustment disorder with prominent features of depression at the time of the killing'. The sentence was reduced to 12 months' imprisonment suspended for 12 months.

What is not clear is, in relation to doing what specific thing or things was the appellant's ability substantially impaired. It might have been the ability to form a rational judgement or it might have been the ability to exercise self-control. However, given the psychiatric evidence that the appellant appeared to have been 'an individual who has not easily recognized his emotional distress', it might even have been the ability to understand the nature of his own conduct.

Commenting on this case, Clough (2015) (19) observes:

> A plea of manslaughter by reason of diminished responsibility was accepted, based *only* on a diagnosis of 'adjustment disorder', with the psychiatric report reading that the defendant had not recognised his 'emotional distress' in the circumstances (my italics).

The word 'only' suggests some scepticism about the acceptance of emotional distress and such a minor disorder as the basis for a diminished responsibility plea. The outcome might have been quite different if the psychiatric evidence had been contested or if the defendant did not attract such sympathy, as Mr Webb probably did.

Mr Webb's case is therefore in contrast with that of *R v Douglas* (20), where the defendant went to her parents' house as usual to cook their Sunday lunch. In the course of doing so she drank a significant quantity of wine, achieving a blood-alcohol concentration in the region of three to three-and-a-half times the legal limit for driving. Her mother was 73 years old and of failing health, and suffering from emphysema and long-standing heart disease. She then killed her mother by smothering her with a pillow because, she said, she could not bear watching her being ill. There was conflicting medical evidence before the jury as to the defendant's mental health. The opinion of the defence's psychiatrist was that at the time of the offence she was suffering from an AD as a consequence of her failing to come to terms with the deteriorating health of her mother. It was not disputed that such a disorder, if it existed, was recognized by ICD-10 (21). The view of the defence's psychiatrist was that this was an abnormality of mental functioning that substantially affected the defendant's ability to exercise self-control. The Crown's psychiatrist, in contrast, was of the opinion that this was not a case of AD, but rather, normal distress caused by the defendant's intoxication with alcohol together with normal emotional distress arising out of the difficult domestic situation which she faced:

> This homicide relates to normal emotions; namely the distress that Angela Douglas experienced in seeing her mother's physical illness and decline. In a state of emotional distress, but not mental disorder, and while intoxicated with alcohol, she killed her mother.

Both doctors agreed that the defendant did not cope well with her stress and used alcohol as a means to alleviate stress. The defendant was convicted of murder, and in sentencing her to the mandatory life imprisonment the judge said that the setting of the minimum term to be served had to be approached on the basis that her degree of culpability was lowered by 'a degree of mental disorder falling short of a nature required by law to establish that defence to the charge of murder'. It is therefore clear that, although the defence of diminished responsibility was not made out, the judge accepted that an AD does represent a degree of mental disorder.

The case of *R v Brown* (22) is another example of the successful reliance on a diagnosis of AD as the basis for a diminished responsibility defence. Mr Brown was involved in acrimonious divorce proceedings, and he believed that his wife was trying to manipulate the legal proceedings to increase the costs so that he would end up with as little money as possible. He also claimed that she wanted to deprive him of any real say in their children's education. At the end of a half-term holiday during which the children stayed with him, he secreted a hammer in the bag with his daughter's homework. Upon returning the children to their mother, he then repeatedly and violently struck her with the hammer on 14 occasions. He put his wife, who was by then unconscious, and might by then have been dead, in the boot of the car and, taking the children as well, drove to his own house where he left the children with his girlfriend. He then drove to a remote location where he put the body in a garden box which he then buried in a grave. He had made the arrangements for digging the grave and providing the box before the attack on his wife. A psychiatrist called by the defence was of the opinion that he had developed an AD as a consequence of a number of stressful life events. His evidence was that 'as a result of the pressures which the appellant was under, his ability to exercise self-control at the time of the killing and his acts in disposing of the body were substantially impaired'. A psychiatrist instructed by the prosecution rejected the diagnosis of AD or indeed any other form of mental disorder that amounted to an abnormality of functioning. He suggested that 'in any event if he did suffer from such a disorder, its extent would only be of any relevance if the jury concluded that the defendant had killed his wife without any pre-meditation'. On sentencing Mr Brown to 24 years' imprisonment for manslaughter, the trial judge observed that 'adjustment disorder was a mild disorder which rarely led to violence' and that 'the disorder appeared to have disappeared almost immediately after the killing'. In rejecting his appeal against the sentence, the Court approved of the trial judge's conclusion that Mr Brown 'retained real culpability' for what he had done, and it observed that there was 'no lack of self-control in the appellant's journey to his home, leaving his children there, and then setting off in his controlled endeavours to escape the consequences of what he had done'.

Notwithstanding Clough's scepticism about AD following the case of *Webb*, in the case of *R v Blackman* [2017] EWCA Crim 190, the court accepted that, when Sgt Blackman killed a severely wounded Taliban insurgent in Afghanistan, he was suffering from an adjust-ment disorder—and, according to the psychiatric evidence, an adjust-ment disorder of moderate severity. The court heard evidence: that Sgt Blackman was, in particular, deprived of sleep, which might have led to diminished decision-making capacity; that there was a heightened threat of an attack which affected his cognitive functioning and deci-sion-making; that he may have been in a state of increased arousal as the finding of an insurgent with a high explosive grenade may have triggered a memory of a recent attack when grenades were thrown at the patrol; that he was a 'husk of his former self', and his mood was flat, or had recently been so; that he had been hypervigilant when walking in the countryside in the UK as a result of the need to be alert about improvised explosive devices; that he had become withdrawn, isolative, and increasingly irritable; that he had exhibited an increased startle response in response to a loud bang in a theatre in New York; and that, in contrast to previously, he did no more than was necessary as a commander. The court accepted the unanimous psychiatric evidence that, in the circumstances of this case, the AD substantially impaired Sgt Blackman's ability to form a rational judgement, and it also substantially impaired his ability to exercise self-control. Importantly also, the court recognized that someone with an AD can appear to behave rationally—in this case, moving the body out of sight of a camera, waiting for a helicopter to move away, and stating that he was not to be shot in the head—but nevertheless being at the same time unable to form a rational judgement about the need to adhere to standards and the moral compass set by HM Armed Forces and putting together the consequences to himself and others of the individual actions he was about to take.

In *R v Zebedee* (23), the case of a man who killed his 94-year-old father, who was suffering from dementia, a defence of diminished responsibility based on AD was also rejected by the jury, but it became an issue on sentencing. The appellant's defence at trial was diminished responsibility and/or loss of control. Those defences were supported by evidence from a consultant forensic psychiatrist. His view was that the appellant had developed an AD as a consequence of failing to come to terms with sexual abuse suffered at the hands of his father as a child. The increasing pressure and stress the appellant was under may have impaired his ability to exercise self-control at the time of the killing, disinhibited by the alcohol that he had consumed. The appellant had told the psychiatrist that he believed he had cracked under the pressure. Overwhelmed with a flood of conflicting emotions and in a state of depression and exhaustion, he had lost his self-control. It is worthy of mention that this psychiatrist's evidence was that he thought the burden of caring for Mr Zebedee was really too much for the family as a whole. The psychiatrist called by the Crown disagreed fundamentally. His evidence was that any AD would have manifested itself soon after the alleged abuse, which had apparently ended at least 45 years earlier, and would have persisted only for a matter of months. In his opinion there was no abnormality of mental functioning from a recognized mental condition. The defences of diminished responsibility and loss of control were both left to the jury, but rejected. On appeal, it was argued—successfully—that the judge had failed to reflect sufficiently on, *inter alia*, the matter of 'the appellant's mental state and personality disorder [*sic*]² falling short of diminished responsibility', and the minimum term of the life imprisonment sentence to be served was reduced from 14 to 10 years.

In Scotland, successful mitigation on the grounds of diminished responsibility reduces the offence of murder to culpable homicide. The case of *NYK* (24) is that of a man who was charged with the murder of his wife. At his first trial he was convicted of murder, but at a retrial in 2011, which was ordered after a successful appeal based on the judge's misdirection of the jury, he succeeded with what was then the common law defence of diminished responsibility. Evidence was led from three psychiatrists. One concluded that the petitioner was not suffering from diminished responsibility at the time of the offence. The other two were of the view that, at the material time, the petitioner was suffering from an AD, which had the effect of diminishing his responsibility. It is not clear from the judgement, which concerns an appeal against sentence, how precisely it was asserted that the AD had the effect of diminishing the petitioner's responsibility.

There is now a statutory basis for the defence of diminished responsibility in Scotland. Section 168 of the Criminal Justice and Licensing (Scotland) Act 2010, implemented in June 2012, has abolished the common law defence of diminished responsibility by amending the Criminal Procedure (Scotland) Act 1995, and the defence is made out when the 'ability to determine or control conduct (is) substantially impaired by reason of abnormality of mind', which includes 'mental disorder'.

In Scotland, it would therefore appear that if AD is accepted as a mental disorder, it may successfully reduce murder to culpable homicide if it can be shown that it has substantially impaired the ability to determine or control conduct.

Infanticide

Case law sheds little light on the potential for a diagnosis of AD to be used in support of a defence of infanticide. In order for the defence

---

² There was no evidence of *personality* disorder and this was probably an error in the drafting of the grounds for appeal.

to be successful, under Section 1 of the Infanticide Act 1938 (as amended by s 57 of the Criminal Justice Act 2009), there has to be evidence that, at the time of the act or omission, the woman's 'balance of ... mind was disturbed by reason of her not having fully recovered from the effect of giving birth to the child'. What this means is elucidated by the case of *R v Sainsbury* (25), where the court used the phrase 'left the balance of your mind disturbed so as to prevent rational judgment and decision'. So it would appear that a successful defence would depend on the AD affecting rational judgement and decision-making. High as this hurdle might therefore appear to be, the defence has been accepted in a case where the only abnormality was 'emotional disturbance' (26). Moreover, in a series of cases reported by d'Orbán (27), a half were not suffering from any identifiable mental disorder, and Bluglass (28) has reported one case in which there was no persisting psychiatric disorder other than the woman's distressed state after the homicide, and one in which a woman who gave birth to a baby with Down syndrome manifested nothing more abnormal than shock, inability to accept the appearance of the baby, and hopelessness for the future. These cases, some of which might have attracted a diagnosis of AD, bear out the observation of d'Orbán that, for infanticide, 'the degree of abnormality is much less than that required to substantiate "abnormality of mind" amounting to substantially diminished responsibility'. Thus, an AD insufficient to found a defence of diminished responsibility may be sufficient to found a defence of infanticide.

Practical implications

Box 12.1 sets out an approach in cases where the diagnosis of adjustment is an issue. It is important to remember that the duty of the expert is to provide independent and impartial evidence that assists in the administration of justice. The expert who tailors his evidence to suit the party instructing, and probably paying, him or her (handsomely, they hope) runs the risk of damaging their credibility, and more importantly, obstructing the administration of justice. Adopting the approach in Box 12.1 will not necessarily prevent the psychiatric expert undergoing a difficult cross-examination, but it may assist the court in narrowing and clarifying the issues.

Box 12.1 A framework for medico-legal reporting in cases of alleged adjustment disorder

Describe adjustment disorders as they are described in ICD-10/ICD-11 and DSM-5, drawing attention to differences in approach—specifically, the requirement for functional impairment.

Draw attention to the caution that both ICD and DSM require when using their classifications in legal settings.

Explain that DSM-5 regards adjustment disorders as subthreshold conditions, whereas ICD-10 does not and ICD-11 probably will not.

Point out that there are no universally agreed diagnostic criteria and that although diagnosis depends on clinical judgement, this is a valid process.

If you rely on criteria for research, be prepared to justify your reliance on them in preference to guidelines for application in the clinical setting.

Point out that there is a real difficulty in that, in distinguishing adjustment disorders from normal reactions to adverse events or circumstances ('stress'), there is insufficient research evidence concerning normal responses to specific types of adversity.

Acknowledge that, notwithstanding what may be agreement as to the diagnosis of AD, psychiatrists may disagree for genuine reasons as to whether or not an AD amounts to a recognizable psychiatric illness or mental disorder.

Analyze the symptomatology and any effects so as to be able to explain why the diagnosis of AD is, or is not, made out.

Explain how the symptomatology does, or does not, satisfy the legal definitions (e.g. psychiatric injury, nervous shock, abnormality of mind, mental disorder) or legal criteria (e.g. substantial impairment of mental responsibility, ability to determine or control conduct).

Set out, and be able to justify the reliance on, such research as may assist the court, such as the evidence associating a diagnosis of AD with risk of deliberate self-harm and suicide and the evidence as to the severity of symptomatology in AD compared with that in major depressive disorder.

References

1. *R (on the application of B) v Dr SS, Responsible Medical Officer and Others* [2005] EWHC 1936

2. Judicial College. Guidelines for the assessment of general damages in personal injury cases. Oxford: Oxford University Press; 2015.

3. **Rix KJB, Cory-Wright C.** How shocking: compensating secondary victims for psychiatric injury. BJPsych Adv. 2018; in press.

4. *Jaensch v Coffey* (1984) 155 CLR 549

5. *McLoughlin v O'Brian* [1983] 1 AC 410

6. **Mullany N, Handford P.** Mullany & Handford's tort liability for psychiatric damage. 2nd ed. Law Book Co of Australasia; 2006.

7. **Rix K.** Expert psychiatric evidence. RCPsych Publications; 2011.

8. County Court (Newcastle upon Tyne), 13 December 2013 (unreported)

9. *McCarroll v Northern Ireland Housing Executive* [2012] NIQB 83

10. *Webb v Norfolk & Norwich University Hospital NHS Trust* [2011] EWHC 3769 (QB)

11. *Tarakhil v The Home Office* [2015] EWHC 2845 (QB)

12. *Manzi v King's College Hospital NHS Foundation Trust* [2016] EWHC 1190 (QB)

13. **Bachem R, Casey P.** Adjustment disorder: A diagnosis whose time has come. J Affect Disord. **227**:243–53.

14. *R v Hayes* [2015] EWCA Crim 1944

15. *R v Moffat* [2014] EWCA Crim 332

16. *R v Byrne* [1960] 2 QB 396

17. *HM Advocate v Savage* (1923) JC 49

18. *R v Webb* [2011] EWCA Crim 152

19. **Clough, A.** J. Crim. L. 2015, 79(5), 358–72

20. *R v Douglas* [2014] EWCA Crim 2322

21. World Health Organization. The ICD-10 classification of mental and behavioural disorders. Geneva: World Health Organization; 1992.

22. *R v Brown* [2011] EWCA Crim 2796

23. *R v Zebedee* [2012] EWCA Crim 1428

24. *NYK* [2013] CSOH 84

25. *R v Sainsbury* (1989) 11 Cr App R (S) 533

26. **Mackay RD.** The consequences of killing very young children. Crim Law Rev. 1993;**40**:21–30.

27. **d'Orbán P.** Women who kill their children. Br J Psychiatry. 1979;**134**:560–71.

28. **Bluglass R.** Infanticide and filicide. In: Bluglass R, Bowden P, editors. Principles and practice of forensic psychiatry. Churchill Livingstone; 1990. p. 523–8.

Index

Tables and boxes and indicated by an italic *t* or *b* following the page number.